CROHN'S AND COLITIS
THE FLARE STOPPER™ SYSTEM.

A Step-by-Step guide
based on 30 years of Medical Research
and Clinical Experience

Galina Kotlyar, MS RD LDN

BALBOA.PRESS
A DIVISION OF HAY HOUSE

Balboa Press books may be ordered through booksellers or by contacting:

Balboa Press
A Division of Hay House
1663 Liberty Drive
Bloomington, IN 47403
www.balboapress.com
844-682-1282

Print information available on the last page.

ISBN: 978-1-9822-7555-6 (sc)
ISBN: 978-1-9822-7554-9 (hc)
ISBN: 978-1-9822-7556-3 (e)

Library of Congress Control Number: 2021920880

Balboa Press rev. date: 01/06/2022

Disclaimer for the Book

The Information and content provided in this book is for educational purposes only and is not meant to substitute the advice provided by your own physician or any other medical professional. You should not use the information contained in this book for self-diagnoses or self-treatment of a disease.

The statements and products in this book have not been evaluated by the United States Food and Drug Administration (FDA) and are not intended to diagnose, cure, treat or prevent any disease. You should not use the information contained in this book for diagnosing and/or treating a disease. Anyone suffering from any illness should consult a health care professional.

This book describes the opinions and experiences of the author. The author shall have neither liability nor responsibility to any entity or any person to any damage, loss, or injury caused directly or indirectly by the information contained herein. The author is not a doctor, nor does she claim to be. She is a registered and licensed dietitian/nutritionist. Please consult your own physician before beginning any program including the program described in this book. If you fail to do so, you are acting at your own risk. If you choose to use the information on www. knowyourgut.com and in this book, you agree to defend, indemnify, and hold harmless Balboa Press, knowyourgut.com and the author of this book from all claims, expenses, of any nature whatsoever (including attorney's fees (for which Balboa Press, knowyourgut.com and the author may become liable resulting form the use or misuse of any information or any products sold through www. knowyourgut.com website.

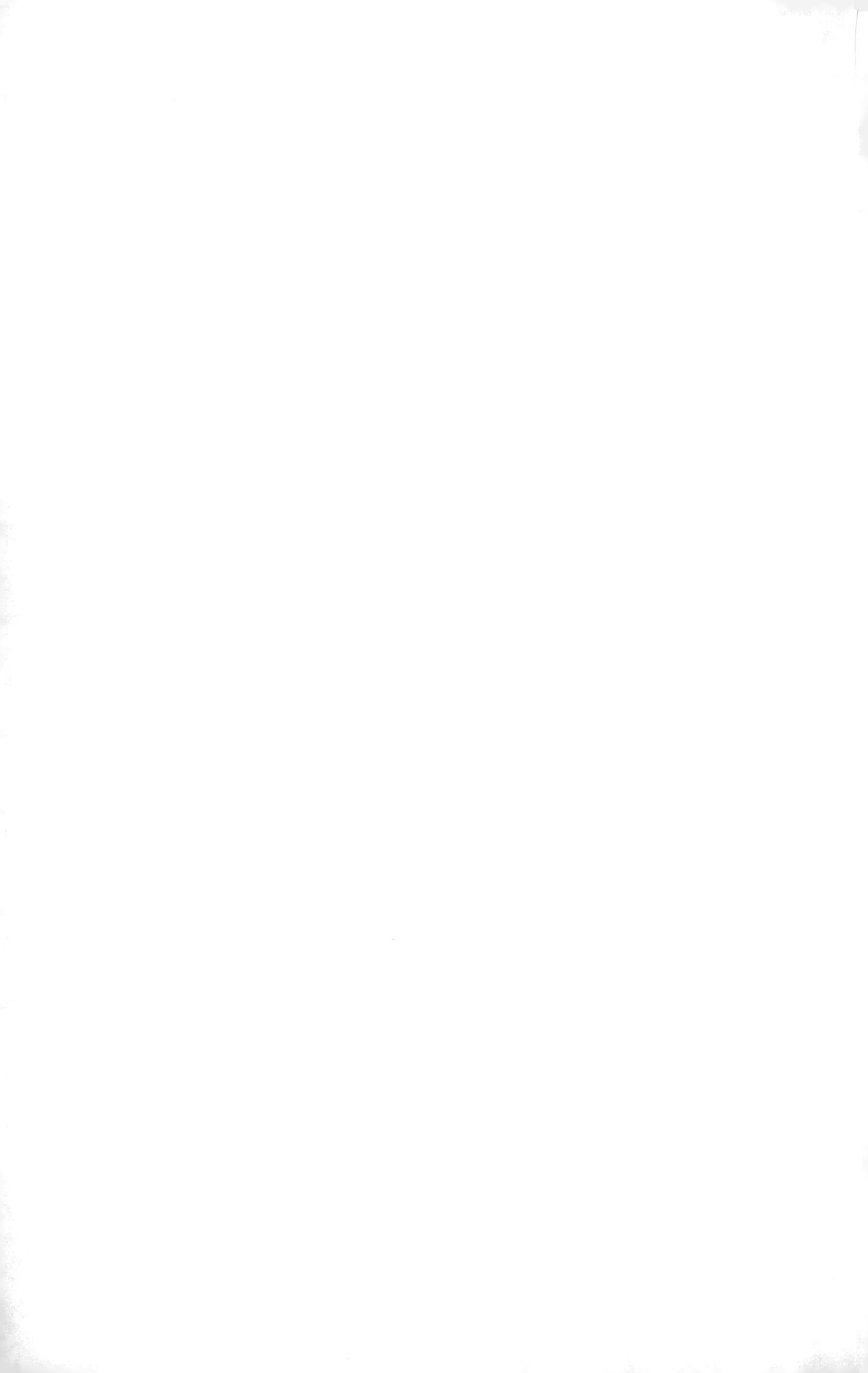

CONTENTS

PROLOGUE

Do you have ulcerative colitis or Crohn's disease?
Have your medications & supplements stopped working for you?
You are not alone.

In 1979, I was diagnosed with ulcerative colitis. Over the years, all the prescribed medications stopped working on me. Anti-inflammatories, antifungals, steroids, antibiotics - all eventually failed.

I continued to live in constant pain, bleeding profusely, losing weight, feeling life itself flowing out of me, with every drop of blood I lost. I thought I was unlucky, a freak, an anomaly. So, I continued to beg my doctors for a new, better medication, but every new medication given to me was eventually failing.

When my doctors finally acknowledged that no medication worked on me anymore, I was totally devastated. They offered me the only option left in their arsenal - the most radical surgery called "full colectomy", where the entire colon (large intestine) is removed. (More on this in the chapter "My IBD story: from dying to living").

Their reasoning was: no colon = no colitis = cure.

I was physically exhausted by years of constant pain, continuous bloody diarrhea, debilitating fatigue, and severe weight loss. However,

I maintained my capacity for critical thinking. The doctor's reasoning for the surgery did not sit well with me.

I didn't see the logic of removing an entire vital organ and calling it a colitis "cure".

My thinking was simple: If my colon was healthy once and then became diseased, there should be a way to fix it, not just cut it out. Would you cut your head off if you had a headache?

So, against my doctors' advice, and to their complete surprise, I refused surgery. I still remember having only one recurring thought: "There must be a better way…There must be a better way…There must be a better way…"

My doctors, having no other options to offer, gave up on me. But I didn't give up on myself. I decided to find a better way to stop my suffering… to find a way to keep my beloved colon, or…die trying.

As you may have guessed by now - I didn't die.

For 30 years, I searched for knowledge on how to deal with this chronic debilitating disease. My own suffering with IBD motivated my scientific research and professional clinical experience as a holistic nutritionist in a very personal way.

I found a way to heal myself.

This is how The Flare Stopper™ System was born; I created it to share my knowledge with my fellow IBD sufferers.

The System worked not only for me but for many of my clients that I've worked with in my clinical practice.

Later in this book, you'll find the whole story of my sickness and recovery.

Yes, RECOVERY. And that is FULL RECOVERY from this so-called "incurable" sickness. It took many years, plenty of suffering, painful mistakes, and a ton of money.

Happily, I am now totally cured. And I know: if I did it, so can you.

This book is for those like me, and the many clients of mine, who stopped responding to medications. This book is for those who might feel like they're at the end of their rope.

Believe me, I know how it feels when you're not living, but rather, existing day to day... in seemingly endless pain and debilitating fatigue during disease flare-ups. Or, during those ever-shrinking remissions, living in anxiety and fear of not knowing when your next flare will strike. And when it does, I know what it's like to feel completely hopeless and horrified, realizing that your next "best" medication does not work for you anymore. Oh, I know how it feels, my friend.

Life may seem very dark to you right now.

But I am here to show you the way to healing. As both a patient and a healthcare professional, I'm in a unique position to understand your pain and struggle. If you are anything like me, seeking an alternative and natural way to heal yourself, this book is for you.

Conventional medicine couldn't heal my IBD; this is more common than you think.

I discovered the statistics about the glaring inefficiency of conventional treatments for IBD.

Here are 3 shocking facts, as described by the highly regarded Mayo Clinic:

1. More than 33% of patients with ulcerative colitis and Crohn's disease will not respond to initial drug therapy, and about **60% of people who initially respond to drug therapy stop responding over time.**[1]

2. A certain number of people with ulcerative colitis **develop a reaction to sulfasalazine and mesalamine, which results in worsening of colitis related symptoms, including more diarrhea, bleeding, and weight loss.**[2]
3. Patients who fail to respond to medications may develop intestinal fibrosis, which can result in stricture formation. **Over 50% of Crohn's disease patients have intestinal obstruction during their life, which often requires surgery. Up to 30% of patients with ulcerative colitis will require surgery over their lifetime.**[3]

But know this now – these grim statistics don't have to be your fate.

Full restoration of healthy gut function and a flourishing life can be yours.

I spent many years learning how to stop my colitis flares and the flares of my IBD clients.

THERE IS A WAY. DO NOT GIVE UP!

COMPLETE RECOVERY IS POSSIBLE!

My dear friend, for me your pain is PERSONAL.

That is why I bring this vital knowledge to you, with a feeling of genuine empathy.

I created this book as a complete guide to stopping your flares, once and for all. Use the knowledge and the tools in this book to get well.

I know what it takes; let me guide you to it.
You just need your will and discipline to follow.
Vibrant health is within your reach now.

With love and deepest compassion,
Galina

References

[1] https://www.mayoclinic.org/es-es/medical-professionals/digestive-diseases/news/managing-refractory-ibd/mac-20430383

[2] https://www.mayoclinic.org/es-es/medical-professionals/digestive-diseases/news/managing-refractory-ibd/mac-20430383

[3] https://www.mayoclinic.org/es-es/medical-professionals/digestive-diseases/news/managing-refractory-ibd/mac-20430383

INTRODUCTION

This book is a tested PRACTICAL GUIDE to effectively stopping IBD flare-ups.

In this book, you will learn:

- How to quickly stop bleeding, diarrhea, and cramps
- How to remove hidden triggers of IBD symptoms
- How to remedy malnutrition by improving absorption of nutrients
- Simple, effective, life-saving tips and modalities never discussed before for ultimate gut healing of Crohn's Disease and ulcerative colitis.

The principles of The Flare Stopper™ System are backed by numerous scientific studies conducted by world-class medical research facilities and doctors. You will see references to various scientific studies all along the way.

More broadly, this book is an introduction to a new evidence-based approach that challenges the current official position of the medical establishment regarding IBD being an "incurable autoimmune" disease.

The Flare Stopper System has been successful for me, as well as for those who followed my nutritional guidance in their quest to regain their intestinal health. You can see my patients' testimonials at knowyourgut.com/testimonials.

Who am I and why should you trust me?

I am Galina Kotlyar, MS RD LDN, a holistic health professional with over 30 years of research, practice, and clinical experience in advising patients with ulcerative colitis and Crohn's disease.

"So what?", you may say... "The internet is full of well-educated health professionals claiming similar expertise".

And you would be right, except this is not ALL that I am.

I am also a fully recovered ulcerative colitis patient.

Once again, so it can really sink in with you:

Yes, I am a FULLY RECOVERED ulcerative colitis (UC) patient.

Why is being a fully recovered UC patient a big deal?

It's a big deal because, according to the MedicineNet definition, ulcerative colitis "is a lifelong illness with no specific cause or cure."[1]

I suffered for years from the most severe form of colitis, ulcerative pancolitis. Here is an opinion about ulcerative pancolitis from ibdrelief.com: "ulcerative pancolitis is a life-long chronic condition which cannot currently be cured."[2]

But I can tell you...I did what conventional medicine thought was impossible.

I cured my "incurable disease" through continuous research and application of a Flare Stopper™ diet and innovative therapies. I transformed myself - from a statistically hopeless UC patient into a happy and healthy woman.

Today, I can live the healthy, fulfilling life I was destined to live. I no longer fear colitis flares. And finally, I have strength and energy to do the physical activities I enjoy so much: yoga, belly dancing, weight training, and swimming in the ocean.

Now, let me tell you about my clinical experience and success stories.

Clinical Experience

For over 30 years, I've worked in hospitals, nursing homes, and in my own private practice. I've seen thousands of clients over the years, from all walks of life, from newborns to 95-year-olds.

As a clinical nutritionist and registered dietician, I've encountered people with a wide variety of health issues: digestive, cardiovascular, metabolic, psychiatric, and others. In my work, I observed how the systems of the body were interlinked. I saw how diet and lifestyle modifications could restore health and vitality, even in the elderly and sick.

In my private practice, I helped many ulcerative colitis and Crohn's clients go from horrible flares to fully restored digestive function. I believe that digestive health is the basis for a healthy body.

I give my clients the unique knowledge and practical tools needed to help them achieve fast and long-lasting remission. And I tested all these healing modalities on myself first. I assure you; I didn't do this simply out of my own professional curiosity. Far from it. I did it out of desperate necessity when I was fighting for my life, trying to stop my own ulcerative colitis nightmare.

This knowledge didn't come easy to me - rather, it was the result of years of painful trials and errors experimenting on myself, and exhausting search for new answers. I wanted to find something that worked not only for me, but for others as well.

My colitis case was very severe and stubborn. It lasted years. Early on in my disease, I stopped responding to all known medications. At times,

I was literally fighting for my life, desperate for help, but traditional medicine had nothing to offer me except radical surgery.

Stubbornly clinging to life, I kept on searching around the world for relief to my suffering. As a traditionally educated and clinically trained healthcare professional, I knew how to dive deep into research. I read independent scientific studies, conducted by world-class medical institutions. Through thick and thin, I experimented with many new remedies, foods, and modalities.

I needed to find scientific proof of my empirical findings before I could recommend them to others, no matter how well those discoveries worked for me.

My Mission

My life's mission is to help you to get well in the shortest time possible without spending thousands of dollars on treatments, diets, and supplements that don't work. This book is the real deal where you can learn the TRUTH about ulcerative colitis and Crohn's disease. The TRUTH will set you free. Free from misinformation and manipulation.

Most importantly, applying the simple and inexpensive healing remedies offered in this book, you will set yourself free of life-long pain, misery, and possible financial devastation. You will acquire the tools necessary to become well, once and for all.

I have successfully implemented this program for myself, and over the years, I've guided many people to do the same. Even the ones who had been sick for years with draining, inflamed fistulas and bloody diarrhea, who stopped responding to the latest treatments modern medicine has to offer... They too fully recovered after completing my program. I have been blessed to witness the remarkable transformation these people experienced. They went from sick, exhausted, depressed, and hopeless to vibrantly healthy, energetic, and happy after completing my program.

Do You Have the Guts To Think Outside Of The Box?

Unfortunately, many people with any form of Inflammatory Bowel Disease (IBD) are clueless about the true causes of their disease. But it's not their fault.

People with IBD are greatly misinformed by the conventional medical community. It's not that those practitioners of Western medicine are purposefully misleading people with IBD - they are simply not sufficiently trained in cause-related, or preventative medicine. Instead, they are trained to relieve symptoms.

Sadly, the only tools at their disposal are pharmaceutical drugs and surgeries. Unfortunately, most of their patients simply don't know (at least at the beginning), how ineffective, damaging, and painful conventional medical treatments can be. Patients are told by their doctors that drugs and surgery are their only options.

Well, this is NOT the whole truth.

In this book, you will be getting the WHOLE truth, as I see it at this time in my journey. The solution to healing IBD lies neither solely in conventional medicine, nor solely in alternative medicine. Both systems have things to teach us and things that can help. You must understand the correct application of each of these methods, depending on where you are with your disease.

One thing is for sure: the road to recovery will be different for each person.

However, the basic principles are the same, as you'll see in later chapters. Moreover, I never recommend anything to others that I haven't tried on myself first. This allows me to relate to my patients in a very powerful way. I know your pain, I understand your struggle, and I know what it takes to heal.

Success Stories

Here are some stories from my patients who had the guts to THINK and ACT outside of the box. They had both discipline and determination to get well. They completed my system in full.

Testimonial #1: Lauren, Crohn's Disease patient

> "I have been diagnosed with Crohn's disease 12 years ago and since then I have continuously experienced painful symptoms. About 10 years ago I developed three (3) anorectal fistulas that continuously leaked pus and blood with continuous painful inflammation around the fistulas. I have undergone multiple surgeries resulting in 2 (two) setons being surgically placed in my anorectal area to ensure adequate drainage of pus and blood. Since then, the fistulas continued to drain pus and blood with various degrees of inflammation, swelling, burning and pain around the setons.
>
> Additionally, I have experienced continuous chronic inflammation in the small intestine, inflamed hemorrhoids, and chronic sinus headaches.
>
> In addition to being treated by my medical doctors, I have tried different diets, and I was taking a total of 32 various supplements a day. Despite my best efforts with diet and supplements, I continued to suffer from small intestine inflammation and constantly draining and painful perianal fistulas.
>
> In July 2017 remaining in the above-described condition, I engaged the services of Galina Kotlyar. After completing her program, I felt healthy. Nevertheless, I have decided to consult with my GI doctors to obtain objective confirmation of my recovery.

My new MRI test and my new colonoscopy that followed has indicated that my 'Crohn's disease of the small bowel and colon is in full remission'. Also, according to the doctors 'the skin around the seton looked healthy, and there was no drainage'. So, both my setons were removed, and my doctors congratulated me and confirmed my 'full remission' and a complete healing of my intestines.

Now, I feel like a new person. I am free from debilitating pain, suffering and constant wound care. I can sit on my office chair without pain in my butt and without using a special pillow. I feel like a new woman. I can wear my bathing suit without worrying about fistula drainage.

Finally, I am ready to become a mom. No more being debilitated with feelings of fear and powerlessness. The knowledge I have acquired through Galina's program has put me back in control of my health, my life and my future."

- Lauren C., Madison, Alabama

Testimonial #2: Abhishek, Universal Ulcerative Colitis (aka Pancolitis) patient

"I was diagnosed with Universal Ulcerative Colitis with rectal bleeding, active gastritis, acute proctitis and haemorrhage of rectum and anus, and very low vitamin D level (24ng/mL) in 2017. I was admitted to ER with bloody diarrhoea with mucus up to 5 times/day, stomach pain and urinary infection. Was prescribed CIPRO for urinary infection, plus steroids and Melamine for UC. The steroids and Melamine did not work, so I was given IMURAN (immunosuppressant) together with pain relieving - hydrocodone with acetaminophen.

Nevertheless, my flare with diarrhea and bleeding continued even while I was taking all these medications. The amount of blood I was losing daily was scary, up to 4 tablespoons of blood with every stool passage. My GI doctor told me that there is no cure for universal ulcerative colitis except the surgery whereby my entire colon would be removed. I was devastated with this news.

Introduction to Galina's System:

July 17, 2017. First consultation with Galina. By this time I had lost 8 lbs, and I was already hospitalized twice

July 25th 2017 - began Galina's System.

History of my recovery is as follows:

After 6 days of being on the Program, my diarrhea, mucus and bleeding stopped. The results were nothing short of extraordinary.

I have continued with the program. Stopped all other meds. While following the Program, I learned what to eat and what not to eat for a healthy gut as well as the importance of therapeutic enemas, oxygen therapies and timely ICV adjustments for improving gut immune system.

By March 2018, my blood tests have indicated two major improvements:

-First: vitamin D level has gone up to a new healthy 75.7 ng/ml, a 300% increase in 5 months.

-Second: my blood iron level have improved dramatically, from 16 mcg/dl in October 2017 to 47 mcg/dl, another 300% increase within 5 months period.

This is especially remarkable since I did NOT take any iron supplements while being on Galina's Program, which included, among other modalities, oxygen therapies and Galina's gut restoration protocol.

My new healthy life.

Now I feel happy, healthy and energetic. My stool is well formed with no blood or mucus. I feel in control of my life because Galina gave me the practical knowledge of how to maintain my disease in remission.

Most importantly: my wife and I were planning to have a child, but due to my disease were were afraid to start a family. Now, I feel and look healthy and my tests confirm it. I've gained weight, feel strong and ready to create a healthy baby."

- Abhishek K., Brookfield, Wisconsin

The Flare Stopper™ System

The Flare Stopper System is based on solid scientific research and 30+ years of my personal and clinical experience. Perfecting this system took me a lot of time, trials, and experimentation. There was pain and suffering for me in the process when I tried something that didn't work. And now that I am clear about what works and what doesn't, you don't have to suffer. I know, if you use my experience and practical knowledge, you will radically change your life for the better by regaining control of your body, your life, and your destiny.

Learn the facts and apply the tools provided in this book.

I am telling you here and now: you CAN heal your gut once and for all.

Never give up! Don't settle for a life of pain and misery!

Your health is in your hands now.

In the next chapter, you can read the story of my personal trip into colitis hell - and my journey back to vibrant health.

References

[1] https://www.medicinenet.com/is_ulcerative_colitis_curable/article.htm

[2] https://www.ibdrelief.com/learn/what-is-ibd/what-is-ulcerative-colitis/pan-ulcerative-colitis

CHAPTER 1

My Story: From Dying to Living

LET ME GIVE YOU SOME BACKGROUND ABOUT MYSELF. YOU WILL LEARN why I am so motivated to help you. My ulcerative colitis story is unique, or... maybe not so much. I suppose that is for you to decide.

Coming to America

Back in the late 70s when I was 17, I left my hometown, Odessa, Ukraine with my parents and my little sister. We were overjoyed to begin a new life in the U.S.A.

In the next year, I lived in Brooklyn, New York, attending a college that I liked, and dreamed about my future career in medicine. Everything was going amazing in my new American life.

Getting Sick with Ulcerative Colitis

Things were great - except for one "very annoying" (how I thought of it then), but an extremely debilitating situation; for no apparent reason, I started running to the bathroom 10 or more times a day, with recurrent bloody diarrhea and severe, gut-wrenching cramps.

Being ecstatically happy about my new life, lost in dreams about my happy future, I simply ignored this "little nonsense". I kept on telling myself: "So what...I am a little sick. . .just a little sick. . ."

But this "little nonsense" persisted - it got worse and worse. Turned out, I was not just "a little sick" - I was VERY SICK.

In the next six months, I lost 25 pounds. I felt continuously exhausted; I was in constant pain. By August of 1979, at age 19, my body had been reduced to a weak, sickly shadow of my former healthy self.

I got worse and worse - suffering from a high fever and severe anemia. Finally, I was admitted to the hospital for the first time in my life.

The diagnosis was grim – ulcerative colitis. I simply could not believe it: "ulcerative colitis? Me? How? Where did it come from?"

I kept questioning my doctors. They casually explained to me: "the causes of this disease are unknown", and "it cannot be cured, only managed".

The "cannot be cured" part of the explanation hit me like a ton of bricks. I remember thinking: "Are they really talking about me?"

My UC Treatments and First Pregnancy

My doctors started me on a course of anti-inflammatory drugs. It worked. . .at the beginning. My bleeding slowed down and my continuous liquid diarrhea became less frequent. Within days, I was back home living my life again. However, my colitis medications provided moderate and temporary relief only at the beginning. With continuous use, they became progressively more ineffective.

That same year, I got pregnant with my first child. Throughout my entire pregnancy, I had what they call a "moderate" flare: diarrhea with blood and mucus, 5-7 times a day. Losing blood and strength, I was constantly drained. I pushed myself through basic household chores, but all I wanted to do was stay in bed all day. Battling a combination of colitis flare-ups, diarrhea, morning sickness, chronic fatigue, and depression during pregnancy was exhausting and demoralizing. It was an overwhelmingly difficult time for me.

The only positive thing I remember from this time was giving birth to a healthy baby - a wonderful ray of sunshine in the midst of my struggle.

After I gave birth, my moderate flare turned into a severe flare (diarrhea 10-12 times a day). I was put back on anti-inflammatory & steroid medications because anti-inflammatory medication alone did not work. Nevertheless, I continued running to the bathroom much more than before.

My Story of Wrong Diagnoses

Which colitis is it: ulcerative colitis (UC) or amebic colitis? Wrong diagnoses can be deadly...

At first, when I came to my GI doctor with complaints of bloody diarrhea and abdominal pain, I was given a diagnosis of ulcerative colitis. My doctor prescribed a standard UC treatment of steroids and anti-inflammatory medications. I was quickly sent home with a pep talk instruction: "take your medications diligently and you'll be fine".

Well, diligence is my strong suit, and I was committed to get rid of my debilitating condition. Naturally, I was anticipating a quick and full recovery. Instead, the medication made my condition worse - shockingly worse.

Before the prescribed medications, I ran to the bathroom 5 to 7 times a day. After diligently taking medications, I was forced to practically live in the bathroom.

I began to have bloody diarrhea up to 15 times a day, with more cramps and abdominal pain than ever before.

It was beyond disappointing. Now I was really scared, lost, and anxious. Thus began the second round of my life-long battle with UC. As it turned out, my diagnosis of ulcerative colitis was wrong. VERY wrong. And a wrong diagnosis leads to a wrong treatment. I found this out the hard way.

Instead of ulcerative colitis, it turns out I had amebic colitis, caused by a parasite called entamoeba histolytica. This parasite attaches itself to the intestinal lining and ruptures the walls of intestinal cells, causing deep-tissue inflammation, colon ulceration, and possible invasion of the liver. I was misdiagnosed because the symptoms of ulcerative colitis and amebic colitis are very similar: bloody diarrhea, abdominal pain, anemia, weight loss, fatigue, etc.

I was misdiagnosed twice.

My first GI doctor failed to check me for parasitic infections. He based his diagnoses on the results of my colonoscopy and my symptoms. He assumed that I have ulcerative colitis, ignoring the possibility of amebic colitis.

My second GI doctor ordered testing for parasitic infections, twice. This test is called ova and parasites (O&P). In this test, a lab technician examines a stool sample under a microscope, looking for parasites. Unfortunately, this test often comes back with false negatives for ameba because the non-pathogenic ameba *Entamoeba dispar* morphologically (in form and structure) looks very much like the pathogenic ameba *Entamoeba histolytica* As a result of two negative stool tests and after a full medical assessment of my case, my second doctor also assumed that my symptoms were caused by ulcerative colitis.

Both doctors misdiagnosed me, which led to me being prescribed the wrong medication, worsening my condition.

They treated me with anti-inflammatory medications and steroids, which was standard medical protocol for ulcerative colitis patients at the time. In contrast, amebic colitis is usually treated with antibiotics and anti-parasitic medications.

These medications are staggeringly different. In amebic colitis, steroid medication works like putting gasoline on fire - the ameba parasite uses the steroid to multiply even stronger and faster. That is why my condition got worse.

Years later, I learned that I was not alone in getting sick with amebic colitis. Worldwide, this parasite "annually infects about 50 million people, and can cause amebiasis, which is characterized by bloody diarrhea, colitis and liver abscesses.

As many as 100,000 people die of this disease per year, and 12% of travelers who develop acute diarrhea after returning from the developing world are diagnosed."[1]

After studying my misdiagnosis problem in depth, I learned that administration of corticosteroids during amebic colitis must be avoided at all costs in order to prevent development of fulminant amebic colitis. This finding was confirmed by a systematic review study published in the professional PLOS Journal.[2]

So, what is fulminant amebic colitis?

According to Dr. V.K. Dhawan:

> *"Fulminant amebic colitis is a rare complication of amebic dysentery (< 0.5% of cases). It presents with the rapid onset of severe bloody diarrhea, severe abdominal pain, and evidence of peritonitis and fever. Predisposing factors*

> *for fulminant colitis include poor nutrition, pregnancy, corticosteroid use, and very young age (< 2 years). Intestinal perforation is common. Patients may develop toxic megacolon, which is typically associated with the use of corticosteroids. Mortality from fulminant amebic colitis may exceed 40%. Chronic amebic colitis is clinically similar to inflammatory bowel disease (IBD). Recurrent episodes of bloody diarrhea and vague abdominal discomfort develop in 90% of patients with chronic amebic colitis who have antibodies to E histolytica."*

According to Dr. Vihod K Dhawan:

> *"Amebic colitis should be ruled out before treatment of suspected IBD because corticosteroid therapy worsens amebiasis."* [3]

Finding the Right Doctor

Luckily, I was introduced to a great gastroenterologist, Dr. Alvin Gelb of Beth Israel Medical Center in New York City (NYC). He established the right diagnoses and prescribed the right treatment for me. But it took months to calm down my symptoms to the point that I could resume my normal life.

Dr. Gelb, God bless his soul, is retired now. To this day, I remain eternally grateful to this outstanding professional who established a correct diagnosis and prescribed appropriate treatment for me.

Back then, in the early 1980's, the only laboratory that was able to correctly detect and identify this disease-causing amoeba (E. histolytica) was Jerry Katz's Laboratory for Tropical Medicine in NYC. Dr. Gelb insisted on using only this lab for my correct diagnosis - and rightfully so. The previous tests for ova and parasites, performed by different labs, came back negative. Dr. Gelb saved my life.

Correct Lab Testing is Crucial

This highly pathogenic ameba is a single-cell protozoan parasite, and humans can get infected with it by drinking contaminated water, eating contaminated food, or having contact with people who prepare food and whose hands are contaminated.

Ameba can infect the bowels and the liver, causing frequent watery stools with blood, severe abdominal pain, cramps, fever, fatigue, and weight loss. According to Helio Gastroenterology, "accurate diagnoses of infection with Entamoeba histolytica is difficult" because its appearance under the microscope "is identical to non-pathogenic species called Entamoeba dispar".[1]

New Test for detection of Entamoeba histolytica

Fortunately, almost 40 years later in 2017, the FDA has approved a new test called the "E. Histolytica Quik Chek™" test (developed and manufactured by TECHLAB®). It is a quick and reliable test for detection of Entamoeba histolytica in stool samples "that targets an adhesin protein unique to E. histolytica."[1]

The Right Medical Treatment

Dr. Gelb told me to immediately stop taking steroids and anti-inflammatory medication. Instead, he prescribed antibiotics (Flagyl) and antiprotozoal medication (Iodoquinol), used to treat intestinal infections. And voila! My symptoms started to subside.

The appropriate combination of antibiotic and anti-protozoal/anti-parasitic medication helped arrest my flare and brought me much needed relief from diarrhea, bleeding, and pain. I thought then: "Bingo, I have a miracle drug combo to control my flares!" However, I quickly learned that celebrating my "magic recovery" was premature.

My new fight began - this time, with a yeast infection. Two weeks after I began taking antibiotics, I developed a severe yeast infection with ever-increasing vaginal itching and discharge. Also, I could not eat because I felt nauseous and had no appetite. So, my celebration turned into a realization that my suffering did not stop - it had just transformed itself.

My Life over The Next 8 Years

Despite everything, I continued to believe in conventional medicine and tried to live my life as normally as possible. Life went on. I got divorced, remarried, and had a second child. I continued to believe that if I followed the doctor's protocol exactly, almighty, modern medicine would eventually cure my colitis. I was wrong. VERY WRONG.

Over the next 8 years, I took numerous medications, such as:

- Multiple courses of antibiotics (Flagyl, Cipro, Tetracycline)
- Oral and rectal steroids (Prednisone, Cortenema)
- Anti-inflammatory drugs (Azulfidine)
- Antiprotozoal medication (iodoquinol) for the treatment of a parasitic infection called amebiasis.

Nevertheless, during these 8 years, the vicious cycle repeated like clockwork:

Flare → Medications → Remission →Flare.

Finally, I found myself not responding at all to these medications. Moreover, I had a colonoscopy that was compared to my old colonoscopies. This test revealed that my severe colon inflammation, initially confined to only 20 centimeters (7.8 inches) of the large colon, had now spread to my entire colon.

My doctor's conclusion was that my amebic colitis had become ulcerative pancolitis. And now, I was treated with anti-inflammatory drugs and steroids.

I was receiving the most advanced treatments known at the time, but nothing was working. I continued to bleed and lose weight. I was a prisoner of my illness, not able to travel more than 20 feet from a bathroom at any given time, plagued with bloody diarrhea 15-20 times a day.

At a dead end again?

Being extremely underweight, anemic, progressively weak, and incredibly malnourished, I ended up in the hospital. My digestive tract was so inflamed that I was not able to absorb any nutrients. And so, liquid nutrition was put directly into my bloodstream, through an IV threaded into my vein.

However, even this nourishment didn't last long. Eventually, after 10 days in the hospital, my veins collapsed. And the doctors had to stop my intravenous feedings.

Suddenly, I wasn't able to get any nourishment at all. I couldn't eat. I couldn't drink. I couldn't even get an IV. At this point, I knew I was certainly facing death.

The Last Resort

Because I was not responding to drugs, and my entire colon was inflamed and affected with bleeding ulcers, my doctors wanted to remove my entire colon with surgery. They proposed doing a colectomy (removal of the entire colon, including the rectum). A colectomy would mean spending the rest of my life with a hole in my abdomen, connected to a plastic bag for defecation.

My doctors openly acknowledged that, considering my weak state of health, complications should be expected, and my "recovery" may be "somewhat delayed", without any particular timeline.

I kept on asking my doctors why the disease was worsening, and they kept telling me that "the causes of ulcerative colitis are unknown" and that "symptoms cannot be controlled with drugs anymore". Weary and desperate, I started to consider this drastic surgery.

My doctors also advised me and my family that, due to my frail condition, the risk of death during or after such an invasive surgery "cannot be ruled out". If I survived, my life "with the bag" would require long-term treatments with strong medications that would likely produce serious side effects over time. How's that for a pep talk?

Feeling helpless and exhausted, I wept quietly in my hospital bed. I had hit rock bottom. The thought of suicide suddenly flashed in my head. I was only 29 years old.

My Realization

In the middle of sleepless night, I lay completely exhausted on a hospital pillow wet from my tears. These clear new thoughts appeared:

- I just don't know enough to make a decision.
- My doctors acknowledged that they do not know the true causes of my disease.
- All processes in our world have cause and effect.
- Any disease is a process and ulcerative colitis is no exception to this law. It must have a cause or causes.
- Without eliminating the cause of the disease, it is impossible to eliminate the effects of the disease.
- What if these doctors simply don't know everything, like the ones who misdiagnosed me before?

- The solution is in finding the true causes and eliminating them. If nobody can do it for me, I must do it myself.

This long, logical chain of thoughts appeared in my head as a well-formed concept with one final thought: "Knowledge is Power. I Must Learn More".

I realized that I, and no one else, was ultimately responsible for my health and well-being. Moreover, the thought of my two children growing up motherless changed everything for me. It flipped a switch in my brain. In the next instant, suicide, death, or life as a suffering, disabled invalid were NOT acceptable options. I MUST be there for my kids! I MUST get healthy!

My Decision

I had no more doubts: "This irreversible surgery is NOT for ME. I am too weak to endure such drastic surgery. I could die on the operating table or shortly thereafter. This is my body, and I am responsible for it. I MUST find the true causes of my disease and eliminate them."

In that very moment, my depression and despair transformed into determination to live and be healthy again. I realized that conventional medical doctors, who were desperately trying to help me, could not help me in any way that was acceptable to me. So, I decided to get well on my own, or...well, die trying.

The same day, to the surprise of my doctors, I declined surgery and checked myself out of the hospital, without my family's knowledge. Still dizzy and weak, dressed only in a hospital gown and paper slippers, I stepped out of the hospital lobby hoping to catch a taxi. The usually simple task of catching a cab in the middle of New York City had proven to be a real difficult one for me.

In addition to being dressed only in hospital gown and slippers, I had no money.

This, in combination with my sickly appearance apparently made smart New York cabbies suspicious of my ability to pay, or my sanity... or both. They refused even to stop. Well, not all of them. After seemingly endless number of my attempts to stop a cab, one young gentleman finally stopped and asked me "where to?" I still remember the look on his face when I told him that I needed to go to Brooklyn (a very long ride), and I had no money on me, but my family will pay at the end of the trip.

He just kept on looking at me without answering. His pausing with answer seemed too long for me – he was just another uncaring NY cabby.

Losing my hope, I just stepped away from his car and turned away. And suddenly, he said:

"Hey lady, where are you going? Get in, I'll get you there". Later, during my long ride home he told me that it was something in my eyes that made him do it. I still wonder what it was.

And I still tear up every time when I recall what this fine man done for me on that day.

I still pray for him and his loved ones. God bless him and all the people who can recognize other human being in need and are willing to help. I still believe that people like him make our world beautiful. That is how I delivered myself home that day.

I felt so good walking into my home and coming back to my kids and my husband. I was happy, but still VERY sick. When the initial excitement and tears subsided, the reality struck again.

"Now what?" I thought. That is when my relentless search to heal my body began.

After all, on the day of my "escape" from the hospital, nothing had changed about my health. Moreover, I returned home to the realities and responsibilities of family life. We were an average, middle-class, working family with two young kids. We had bills – lots of bills, including home mortgage, car loan, student loan, and sky-high medical bills. There was so much to take care of. Despite of this, our entire existence revolved around me getting well. And my husband and I soon learned there was no "quick fix" for my condition.

My 30-year search for an IBD cure

My journey to health was like a huge puzzle that I was trying to put together for decades. I was gathering knowledge piece by piece.

In the following years, we spent thousands of dollars on treatments, both conventional and alternative. We used our savings, my parents' savings, and our credit cards. We traveled all over the world, visiting numerous doctors, spas, and clinics in Mexico, Canada, Germany, Bulgaria, Poland, France, and Switzerland.

But no one was able to give me a comprehensive program that would work consistently and ultimately heal my gut. I understood that I had to do it myself.

I spent money, time, and energy. Blood, sweat, and tears. I poured my brain, my heart, and my soul into solving the root cause of my disease. I had God's help, and my family's everlasting love and support.

I decided to dedicate my entire life to the science of holistic medical nutrition therapy and natural healing to heal myself and help others. I spent 8 years doing my undergraduate and graduate degrees in Human and Clinical Nutrition Therapy. I completed an intense internship in clinical nutrition and dietetics at Tulane Medical School, one of the best medical universities in the U.S.

I studied hundreds of scientific journals. I searched for every piece of scientific literature relating to IBD and digestive wellness, over the past hundred years, across different countries and languages. I read original research in English, Russian, and Bulgarian, using my language skills to find whatever knowledge I could get my hands on.

Using scientific research as a clue, I experimented with numerous medications, anti-parasitic herbs, anti-fungal herbs, and hundreds of supplements and liquid meal replacements and therapies. I tried European homeopathy, volcanic minerals, colloidal silver, probiotics, ozone treatments, hydrogen peroxide infusions, vitamin and mineral IVs, chelation therapy, urinotherapy, classical Chinese acupuncture, and much, much more.

You name it, I've done it.

Finally, I've developed the Flare Stopper™ System with principles, remedies and modalities that are not only safe and effective, but also scientifically supported by clinical research of world-class medical facilities and institutions.

In my journey, I helped many IBD people like myself, and had the pleasure of leading them to a bright and healthy future. Repeatedly, I saw the same issues that I had faced, and some that were new to me.

Even though I practice today a naturopathic approach to IBD, I am still a firm believer in the value of classical medical education. While continuing to gather the latest medical research as well as modern and natural health solutions from doctors and healers worldwide, I realized that the REAL solution is not solely in the conventional medical approach; neither is it in the exclusive "all natural" approach. The solution is, in fact, the harmonious marriage of the two.

Most of my breakthroughs, which I define as a combination of therapies and methods that produce the best results, occurred from direct clinical experience with my own healing process and the healing processes of my patients. I remain eternally grateful, with the testimonials of my clients as my best reward.

Learning from Other Healthcare Professionals

While trying to solve my own IBD puzzle, I had many teachers: doctors, scientists, and researchers who I personally met and learned from. I have critically assessed and selected only those concepts and solutions that have been effective, safe, and directly applicable to issues specific to ulcerative colitis and Crohn's disease. Needless to say, I tested all therapies on myself first.

Moreover, we, the IBD people, especially at the time of a flare, are extra sensitive to things we consume and our environment. Therefore, special considerations must be given to those sensitivities. That has been an aim in my Flare Stopper System.

In the end, even though no one had the ultimate solution for me, I gained valuable insights from each doctor. Here are some of the doctors I consulted with, studied with, and learned from:

Dr. Bernard Jensen is known as the father of holistic health. Dr. Jensen practiced his natural therapies for over 60 years. He treated and taught more than 350,000 patients. Dr. Jensen was my beloved teacher. I met him in the late 1980's. He introduced me to an anti-inflammatory bowel restoration program that helped me in my health journey.

He shared his techniques with me, helping me build health and fight my disease. Dr. Jensen sparked my interest in raw vegetable juice fasting, vital broth, therapeutic enemas, and colonics. He introduced me to the ultimate tissue cleansing system for a full restoration of healthy intestinal flora as well as improvement of digestion and absorption of the foods I was eating.

Dr. Robert Atkins of New York was an American cardiologist, known for his popular low-carbohydrate Atkins Diet. I consulted with Dr. Atkins in the 1980's, in his medical clinic on Manhattan's Upper East Side. He introduced me to the idea of food sensitivity tests. He was the first physician who diagnosed me with certain food intolerances.

Dr. Atkins prescribed me a high-protein, high-fat, very low-carb diet, together with a wide array of vitamins, antioxidants, enzymes, and herbs which were supposed to stop my flare. Unfortunately, his supplementation and diet protocol did not stop my flares, but his tests helped me identify and remove foods that my body did not tolerate at the time. This information helped me on my path to digestive wellness.

Dr. Luc De Schepper is an internationally recognized doctor with medical licenses in Belgium and the United States. He is the author of twelve books on holistic health care and known for his success in treating Candida and Chronic Fatigue with diet, supplements, and homeopathy.

Dr. Luc De Schepper was the first physician in the early 1990's who explained to me that healing ileocecal valve inflammation is important when one has IBD and chronic candida infections. Addressing inflammation of my ileocecal valve was instrumental in addressing my small intestinal bacterial overgrowth (SIBO), multiple occurrences of candida infection, and resolving long-standing pain in the lower right quadrant of my abdomen.

Dr. Robert Roundtree is a diplomate of the American Board of Holistic Medicine. In his private practice in Boulder, Colorado, he cares for his patients with a unique combination of traditional family medicine, mind-body therapy, nutrition, and herbology.

Dr. Roundtree explained to me that environmental toxins from heavy metals, drugs, pesticides, and industrial compounds can cause many chronic health conditions, such as immune system depression, chronic fatigue syndrome, recurrent yeast infections, chronic fatigue syndrome, mood swings, fibromyalgia, learning disorders, kidney dysfunction, and even cancer. I learned from him about nutrient-based detoxification therapies that are used to improve the body's ability to excrete toxins. He explained to me that healthy digestion is a must for timely detoxification of environmental toxins, and in the prevention of chronic degenerative diseases. By decreasing toxic load and storage of toxins, affected people can achieve robust health.

Dr. Ronald Hoffman is one of the most famous U.S. practitioners of complementary medicine. He is a founder of the Hoffman Center in New York City. Dr. Hoffman advised me that large doses of Vitamin C and zinc can trigger gastrointestinal distress at the time of IBD flare. That is why, at the time of an acute IBD flare, I don't recommend using vitamins like Vitamin C, B-vitamins, or minerals.

Dr. Hoffman recommended natural botanicals like citrus seed extract instead of antibiotics, as well as L-glutamine and Omega-3 fish oil for nontoxic treatment of ulcerative colitis. For me, he administered intravenous fluids and a "cocktail" of antioxidants, vitamins, and minerals. These treatments helped compensate for the loss of fluids and nutrients I experienced from frequent watery diarrhea during my flares.

Dr. Louis Parrish of New York was a specialist in parasitology. In 1995, Dr. Parrish introduced me to The Protozoal Syndrome (TPS), which describes how "millions of Americans are needlessly suffering from poor health because of protozoal infections", such as Entamoeba histolytica and Giardia lamblia. Dr. Parrish taught me that testing for parasites must always be done in immunocompromised patients. He recommended a rectal swab technique for parasite testing, because his research indicated that a laboratory report from a single stool sample is a false negative 90% of the time.

He advised to begin parasitic treatments with pharmaceuticals, then once the patient's symptoms are stabilized, the further therapy can be done with herbs and supplements.

Dr. Jeffrey Bland is a leader in the field of nutritional medicine. He is known as the "father of Functional Medicine", who founded the Institute for Functional Medicine in 1991.

I met Dr. Jeffrey Bland, Ph.D. in the spring of 1995 at the doctorate seminar at the Foundation for the Advancement in Innovative Medicine in New York. He introduced me to the concept of gastrointestinal restoration through a groundbreaking concept called "The 4R" Gastrointestinal Support Plan: Remove, Replace, Reinoculate, Repair. This Program helps to restore healthy gut functions. Dr. Bland taught me that you cannot heal the gut unless you remove pathogens from the gastrointestinal system first.

Dr. Christo Damianov is a founder of the First Integrative Medical Centre in Sofia, Bulgaria. I had the pleasure of meeting and learning from this outstanding physician and his staff. Dr. Damianov leads the team of doctors that actively uses various treatments in the field of Integrative Oncology. Currently, Dr. Damianov is working on research of IPT treatments, Biomagnetic pairs, as well as immunotherapy, intravenous therapy with high dose of Vitamin C, ozone, laser therapy, electric therapy, etc. for patients with cancer and autoimmune conditions.

FirstLine Therapy (FLT), a new approach to treating disease. I became a certified FirstLine Therapy nutrition educator more than 10 years ago. The FirstLine Therapy approach is unlike today's conventional medical approach. This holistic, science-based treatment plan is designed to identify and correct the true causes of disease by balancing the body's inflammatory response. FLT practitioners provide a clinically designed "therapeutic lifestyle program" that helps people regain health, improve digestion, decrease fatigue, and feel better.

My Life Purpose

For years, my body was my laboratory. I experimented on myself using different remedies and modalities, while I had a chain of seemingly endless colitis flares. It was a process of trial and error - at times very painful, and very expensive. Little by little, with God's help and a lot of gratitude while praying for my life, my tireless experimentations and worldwide research bore fruit. I was able to identify truly effective remedies and modalities that worked on me consistently, and without harmful side effects.

These findings have formed the first foundation of my methodology to stop my flares.

Being a medical professional, prior to recommending any such remedies to others, I had to find independent, scientific and/or medical studies confirming my own findings.

That is why, the Flare Stopper System described in this book includes so many references to independent, scientific and/or medical studies confirming my recommendations.

I encourage you not to skip those references. Knowledge is power. Get convinced and inspired by seeing for yourself what the world-class scientists and medical researchers found about the remedies recommended in this book.

My life purpose is to help people stop IBD flares fast, easy, and effectively, and ultimately heal their bodies completely. Through the years, I continually improved my methods. I want to help others avoid the painful mistakes I made on my road to complete recovery. I want to help as many IBD sufferers as possible. Let me share with you what I have learned.

References

[1] https://www.healio.com/gastroenterology/infection/news/online/%7Bdd342e0a-a837-41e2-b5dc-10825f55f945%7D/fda-clears-rapid-diagnostic-test-for-e-histolytica)

[2] Shirley, Debbie-Ann, and Shannon Moonah. "Fulminant Amebic Colitis after Corticosteroid Therapy: A Systematic Review." *PLoS neglected tropical diseases* vol. 10,7 e0004879. 28 Jul. 2016, doi:10.1371/journal.pntd.0004879

[3] Dhawan, V.K. MD. (2019) "Amebiasis". *Medscape* pp. (1-28)
http://emedicine.medscape.com/article/212029-clinical

CHAPTER 2

What is the real cause of IBD?

THIS CHAPTER WILL HELP YOU UNCOVER THE "HIDDEN" CAUSES THAT most likely contributed to your disease. I call them "hidden" causes because very few health professionals talk about them, while the general population of IBD people remains completely unaware of them. But, this is not their fault. It is not your fault either.

These true causes remain hidden, either because they are known to a very small professional circle of medical scientists, or they are completely lost in the avalanche of information & misinformation on the internet. Regretfully, only a few practicing GI doctors are aware of these hidden causes of IBD.

In this chapter you will learn about the fundamentally different approach I have taken to successful reversing my IBD:

- Conventional Medicine's View of IBD as a disease
  - Causes are unknown
  - IBD is autoimmune disease
  - There is no cure for IBD
- Galina's View of IBD
  - 2 Hidden Causes of Inflammation in IBD
  - IBD is Not Autoimmune Disease
  - Why Most People Get Sick and Stay Sick with IBD

My personal recovery from severe IBD, recovery of those who followed my System and my scientific research indicate that conventional medicine view of IBD disease is INCORRECT.

In this chapter, you will learn how the IBD process usually starts and develops.

Conventional Medicine's View of IBD

The official position of conventional medicine is that the immune system during IBD becomes overactive and starts attacking healthy gut tissue for no good reason. Therefore, they labeled IBD as an autoimmune disease. However, this is simply the description of the IBD process, not the cause. The conventional medical establishment admits they don't know what causes IBD. And because they don't know the cause, they don't know how to fix IBD. They are convinced there is no cure for IBD patients - only management of their disease symptoms. So, conventional medicine manages IBD in two ways: Drugs and Surgeries.

Conventional medicine's treatment plan for IBD is based on the following logic:

Drugs: Suppress symptoms = Suppress the problem

Surgery: Remove the organ = Remove the problem

Now, ask yourself just 2 questions:

1. Can doctors effectively treat disease if they don't know the cause?
2. If the doctors don't know the cause of IBD, why are they telling you there is no cure?

Because conventional medicine marks the root cause of IBD as "unknown", logically for them, the elimination of the root cause is no longer possible. How can you eliminate something that is "unknown" to you?

Following that logic, the current medical treatment model is based solely on suppression of disease symptoms, leaving the "unkown" causes untouched, thereby making a true recovery impossible.

Suppression of the body's normal response is the name of the game

Instead of removing the cause of the patient's inflammation, doctors try to suppress the inflammation with anti-inflammatory medication, and/or suppress the body's immune response with immunosuppressant medication.

The causes of the disease remain. The patient is encouraged to take pharmaceuticals for life, hoping for occasional resolution of symptoms and short-lived remissions. But, this method is doomed to fail. Too many IBD patients have experienced this. This suppression of the disease process causes many additional health problems. Just read up on the side effects of IBD drugs. It's right on the labels, written in black and white by the pharmaceutical companies that manufacture these medications.

The side effects are shocking: abdominal pain, bloody diarrhea, severe bacterial infections, bone fractures, depression, tuberculosis, pneumonia, herpes, multiple sclerosis, congestive heart failure, liver disease, and even cancer. Worsening of symptoms is often blamed on the disease itself (IBD), whereas the worsening could be caused by the drugs the patient is taking.

After a while, IBD patients' quality of life dramatically declines, due to worsening of the disease itself, combined with side effects caused by long-term use of pharmaceuticals. Often patients complain of weight loss, overall body pain, frequent infections, very low energy, disturbed sleep, disappointing sex life, and inability to work.

And if medication does not work, conventional doctors use the ultimate suppression of the disease - surgery. Their idea is to just cut out the diseased intestines and call it a cure. This is especially true in the case of ulcerative colitis.

Can Colon Surgery Cure Colitis?

Since ulcerative colitis is limited to the colon, GI doctors practicing conventional medicine will tell you that the only cure for the disease is colectomy (surgery to remove the entire colon). Believe me, I know these suggestions all too well. Years ago, when my own colitis was labeled "unmanageable", I heard my own doctors suggest these "treatments".

Amazingly, now, decades later, conventional medicine's treatment for colitis remains the same:

NO COLON = NO PROBLEM.

Therefore, many people suffering for years with ulcerative colitis start considering surgical removal of their diseased colon as a final "cure". They hope that after they get rid of their colon, all their digestive problems will be gone. They hope they will be finally cured.

But, what does it mean to be cured?

According to the Merriam-Webster dictionary, the word "cure" means "something (such as a drug or medical treatment) that stops a disease and makes someone healthy again." I fully subscribe to this definition - with emphasis on the words "makes someone healthy again".

The word "cure" means not only elimination of disease symptoms, but also a complete return to optimal health. Unfortunately, removal of your colon does not stop the disease process, and most definitely does not restore your health.

Galina's View of IBD

When I started on my healing journey over 30 years ago, I had to understand why people get sick with colitis and Crohn's in the first place. Here are the facts: ulcerative colitis and Crohn's disease are called Inflammatory Bowel Disease (IBD) for a reason. The reason is: IBD is chronic inflammation of your digestive tract. Let's talk about acute and chronic inflammation.

Acute vs Chronic Inflammation

There are 2 types of inflammation: acute and chronic. Acute inflammation is usually short in duration, and it's a part of a healthy body's normal immune response to infection, toxins, or injury. Some examples of acute inflammation are the flu, the common cold, and hives.

Acute Inflammation

Acute inflammation is not a bad thing. A properly functioning immune system creates acute inflammation as part of the HEALING response. If you cut your finger, your immune system creates acute inflammation in the cut in order to destroy microbes and help repair the damaged tissue. Without acute inflammation, the cut on your finger would never heal. Acute inflammation is a tool your body uses to heal itself, and its presence should be interpreted as a message that something is wrong. Your body creates inflammation when it tries to defend itself against harmful bacteria, viruses, parasites, fungi, and toxins. Therefore, acute inflammation is a normal body response to infection, toxins or injury.

Chronic Inflammation

If pathogens and toxins are not removed, acute inflammation becomes chronic. Chronic inflammation is long in duration, continuous, and relentless. In chronic inflammation, the body's immune system becomes chronically activated or overactive, in attempt to resolve inflammation. If the inflammation is not cleared, the overactive immune system starts breaking down the body's tissues. Examples of chronic inflammation include IBD, arthritis, and lupus.

2 Hidden Causes of Inflammation in IBD

I asked myself a question over and over again: What causes inflammation in IBD?

After years of self-experimentation and clinical research, I understood that there are 2 hidden causes that trigger inflammation in IBD. They are:

1. **Pathogens** (like bacteria, viruses, fungi, parasites)
2. **Toxins** (from drugs, inflammatory foods, environment, stress)

Let's dive into pathogens and toxins that contribute to IBD.

Infection-causing Pathogens may trigger IBD

Studies confirm that both ulcerative colitis and Crohn's disease can be triggered by a specific infectious agent/microorganism, such as pathogenic bacteria, viruses, fungi, or parasites. These harmful bugs can cause chronic inflammation, diarrhea, and abnormal immune response. Symptoms of intestinal infections can be identical to IBD symptoms, such as abdominal pain, fever, bloody diarrhea, and weight loss. These infections can start the IBD disease process and trigger IBD flares. Specific pathogens and infections associated with IBD will be discussed later in this book.

Toxins may trigger IBD

According to Dr. John Coppola, D.C., the founder of San Antonio Neuropathy Center: "Modest estimates have suggested that we are exposed to more than 700,000 different toxic chemicals on a daily basis, and this doesn't include the crazy poisons that GMO companies are pumping into the food supply. According to the Global Healing Center, it isn't abnormal to be exposed to 2,100,000 toxins each and every day."[1]

This avalanche of chemicals contaminates the whole body. Our body absorbs chemicals from food, water, prescription drugs, and personal care products.

The body cannot remove this avalanche of toxic chemicals in a timely manner, which causes a serious build-up of toxins inside various organs and body systems.

The result? Systemic toxicity. People with systemic toxicity often experience damage in the lining of the gastrointestinal tract, which loosens up the tight junctions between the cells of the gut wall. This results in increased intestinal permeability or "leaky gut syndrome", diarrhea/constipation, bloating, gas, fatigue, joint pain, and fungal infections. Unless this flow of toxicity is reduced to a minimum, and your body is purged of accumulated toxins, full recovery and optimum health cannot be achieved. Four types of systemic toxins that may contribute to IBD will be covered in this book.

Here's the good news: once you uncover the true triggers of your IBD, you will finally be able to remove them, allowing your body to heal itself.

So, how do you stop inflammation once and for all? You've probably guessed it by now: get rid of pathogens and toxins, and the inflammation will subside. And with it, your overactive immune system will calm down. These changes will reduce the painful symptoms of your IBD, and your body will start healing.

IBD is NOT an Autoimmune disease

Over 25 years ago, realizing that pathogens and toxins are the root cause of IBD, I finally stopped blaming my sickness on an overactive immune system, genetics, or bad luck. I understood that in IBD, the immune system is attacking infection-producing pathogens and toxins - NOT healthy tissue. Therefore, the concept that the body attacks itself due to a malfunction of your immune system is false.

Pathogens and toxins are the main reasons colitis and Crohn's patients experience chronic activation of the immune system, intestinal inflammation, dysbiosis, and leaky gut. Abdominal pain, bloody diarrhea, impaired digestion, fatigue, and weight loss are simply side effects.

After this realization, I started to look for new solutions to eliminate the REAL causes of my inflammation - pathogens and toxins. In the early 90s, I felt alone on my journey. Back then, it was incredibly rare to meet any medical professional who shared my radical views on the true causes of IBD - the exception was my late teacher Dr. Bernard Jensen.

Happily, sooner or later, the truth becomes obvious. Medical science does not stay still. Finally, my findings from 25 years ago have been confirmed by modern science, which now shows that IBD is not really an autoimmune disease, but really the result of our smart immune system attacking pathogens and toxins. This is what leads to intestinal damage.

WebMD confirmed my decades old findings. Here is their new opinion on IBD - it's a move in the right direction:

> *"The term inflammatory bowel disease (IBD) describes a group of disorders in which the intestines become inflamed. It has often been thought of as an autoimmune disease, but research suggests that the chronic inflammation may not be due to the immune system attacking the body itself. Instead, it is a result of the immune system attacking a harmless virus, bacteria, or food in the gut, causing inflammation that leads to bowel injury."*[2]

So, you should STOP blaming your immune system for its perfectly healthy inflammation response. It's being triggered by pathogens and toxins. The only way to reverse IBD and to heal your gut is to treat the underlying cause of inflammation.

The Process of Getting Sick with IBD

My own recovery, my clinical experience, and the scientific research I have gathered debunks the conventional view of IBD as an autoimmune disease. I began to piece together the story of how IBD happens in the first place. Let's start with the gut lining.

An intact gut lining is the key to a healthy immune system.

The gut wall lining (aka epithelium) works as a barrier between the interior of your gut and your bloodstream. In a healthy person, this intact lining prevents pathogens and toxins from entering the blood, while allowing in water and nutrients. An intact gut lining (mucosa) is interconnected with healthy intestinal flora and a balanced immune system (about 70% of our immune cells reside in our gut). Research consistently indicates that food allergens, pharmaceuticals, toxins, and chronic stress can destroy healthy intestinal flora and damage the delicate gut lining. This destruction of healthy flora, combined with damage in the gut lining, negatively affects our immune system.

How Gut Microbiota Affects Our Immune System

The gut wall lining contains trillions of microorganisms. In a healthy gut, these microorganisms form a community where they coexist in perfect balance: approximately 80% of good bacteria coexist with 20% of bad bacteria. Both good and bad bacteria are needed for healthy digestion. This 80/20 ratio ensures healthy gut function. When this healthy ratio is maintained, the good bacteria is perfectly capable of fighting off harmful bacteria, fungi, and viruses - thereby keeping your gut healthy.

This bacterial community is called gut flora (aka: gut microbiota). Healthy gut flora promotes the integrity of the intestinal lining by forming a protective layer and blocking harmful bacteria.

Furthermore, healthy gut flora is an essential part of the process that converts the food you eat into nutrients necessary for your body to rebuild and regenerate itself. Therefore, healthy gut flora is the foundation of a healthy body and robust immune system. When pathogenic bacteria and yeast species grow out of control, your gut flora becomes disbalanced, creating symptoms of a disturbed gut called *dysbiosis.*

What is Dysbiosis?

"*Dys*" = abnormal, "*Bio*" = life. So, dysbiosis is abnormal life in the gut that results in the breakdown of normal digestion, creating symptoms of indigestion, bloating, abdominal pain, constipation, diarrhea, etc. Inflammatory bowel disease (IBD) is commonly associated with dysbiosis according to Scientists from Soonchunhyang Institute of Medi-Bio Science in Korea.[3]

In dysbiosis, undiagnosed pathogens and hidden toxins accumulate in the gastrointestinal tract. As time goes by, the walls of your intestines become a breeding ground for fungi, parasites, and bacteria. As a result, your gut wall becomes inflamed, loses its integrity, and starts to leak.

The connection between dysbiosis, intestinal barrier destruction (aka leaky gut), and increased susceptibility to disease has been reviewed in September 2017 in Tissue Barriers Journal by scientists from the Department of Immunology, Institute of Biomedical Sciences, University of São Paulo in Brazil.[4]

Leaky Gut in IBD

In a healthy gut, tight junctions between the cells of the gut wall help maintain the integrity of the gut lining. In IBD, dysbiosis and chronic gut wall inflammation cause destruction of these tight junctions between the cells, resulting in increased gut permeability (leakage). The newly formed gaps between the cells allow bacteria, toxins, and incompletely digested food to leak directly into the bloodstream. This condition is known as Leaky Gut or increased intestinal permeability, one of the causes of systemic inflammation.

Systemic Inflammation in IBD

Because of the leaky gut, harmful substances leak into your bloodstream. This triggers an alarm to your immune system. Your body calls on your immunity for help defending against foreign invaders. That is why your immune system "turns on" inflammation and creates antibodies - it's an attempt to get rid of these invaders. But, because of the leaky gut, these harmful substances continue to slip directly into your bloodstream, creating more stress for your already overstressed immune system. Dysbiosis and leaky gut cause continuous activation of the immune system, which results in systemic (whole body) inflammation. That is why, in addition to inflamed intestines, IBD patients may experience inflammation in the eyes, liver bile ducts, and joints.

One thing leads to another. Here's how the process goes:

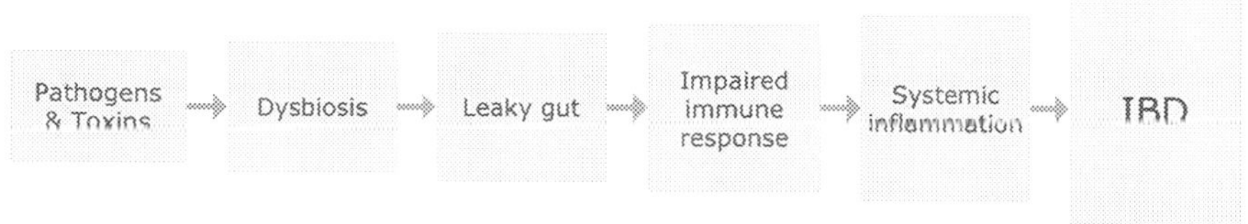
Pathogens & Toxins
Dysbiosis
Leaky gut
Impaired immune response
Systemic inflammation
IBD

Yeast Overgrowth and Fungal Infections are linked to IBD Symptoms

My conventional doctors never talked about the connection between yeast/fungal problems and ulcerative colitis. I learned about it on my own. The first time I learned about the connection of fungal/yeast infection to digestive problems was back in the 1980's, from Dr. William G. Crook's classic book, *The Yeast Connection*.

I devoured the information on how to conquer the devastating effects of yeast overgrowth in my gut. After changing my diet and getting rid of foods laden with sugar and yeast, I noticed a tremendous improvement in my digestive health.

About 20 years ago, I read *The Fungus Link*, written by Doug A. Kaufmann. This book hit home with me because it gave insights on how fungal infection is linked to IBD.

I found the author's suggestions useful in connecting the dots between yeast overgrowth, fungal infection, and IBD symptoms. This book discusses how dysbiosis is caused by antibiotics, poor nutrition, and chemicals. It also confirmed my own empirical findings - those natural antifungals, combined with an anti-candida diet, can help restore digestive health in IBD people.

In 2018, Dr. George A. Stamatiades published a paper, *Fungal infection in patients with inflammatory bowel disease.* They reviewed 14 studies, with data on 1524 patients. "The most common fungal infections in patients with IBD were caused by Candida species (903 infections); the most reported site of Candida infection was the gastrointestinal tract. Available evidence shows that most fungal infections occur within 12 months of IBD treatment and within 6 months when anti-TNFa agents are used."

Also, this study reveals that patients with IBD have increased risk of infections caused by viruses, bacteria, parasites, and fungi, due to use of biologic medications (anti-TNFa), steroids, malnutrition, and surgery.[5]

The Immune System is Trying to Protect Us

Your immune system is the first line of defense against harmful substances trying to enter your body. The immune system's purpose is to identify and eliminate any pathogen or toxin that can make you sick. Pathogens and toxins can destroy healthy intestinal flora and damage the gut lining, creating dysbiosis, leaky gut, and intestinal inflammation.

If pathogens and toxins are not removed, acute inflammation becomes chronic, resulting in dysregulation of the immune system and development of Inflammatory Bowel Disease (IBD). It was eye-opening to see scientific research that confirmed theories I was exploring on myself and in my clinical practice. In the process of doing its job, the immune system becomes overactive while trying to protect the body from pathogens and toxins that cause inflammation and infection.

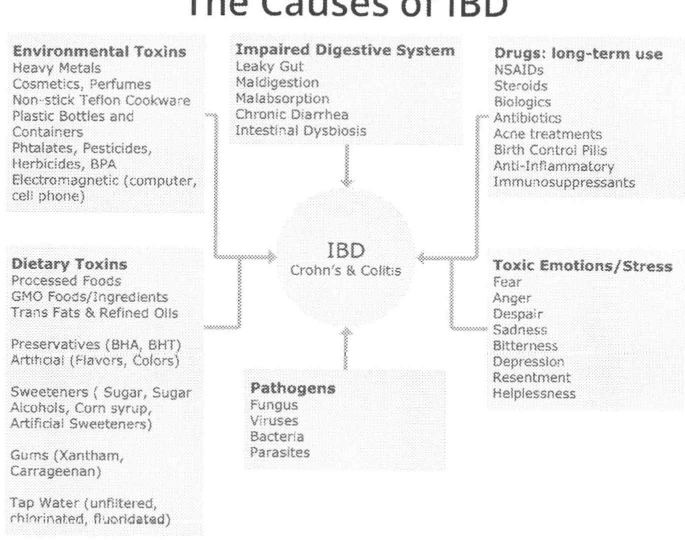

The Flare Stopper System Works

The system in this book works because it properly addresses each reason you got sick in the first place. This system is not just a theory. It's backed up by more than two hundred studies published in medical literature. Just look at the comprehensive list of scientific references in this book.

In the next chapter, we'll learn more about toxins that are present in your drugs, your food, and your environment.

References

[1] https://nervedoctor.info/daily-toxin-intake-how-many-toxins-are-you-accumulating/

[2] https://www.webmd.com/ibd-crohns-disease/inflammatory-bowel-syndrome#1

[3] Lobionda, Stefani et al. "The Role of Gut Microbiota in Intestinal Inflammation with Respect to Diet and Extrinsic Stressors." *Microorganisms* vol. 7,8 271. 19 Aug. 2019, doi:10.3390/microorganisms7080271

[4] Takiishi, Tatiana et al. "Intestinal barrier and gut microbiota: Shaping our immune responses throughout life."
Tissue barriers vol. 5,4 (2017): e1373208. doi:10.1080/21688370.2017.1373208

5 Stamatiades, George A et al. "Fungal infections in patients with inflammatory bowel disease: A systematic review." *Mycoses* vol. 61,6 (2018): 366-376. doi:10.1111/myc.12753

CHAPTER 3

Causes: Toxins. How Various Toxins contribute to IBD

If you are in a flare (a state of constant intestinal inflammation), cleansing your body from toxins is your number one priority. Only after removing toxins and other irritants will your body be able to heal.

If you are serious about stopping a flare and preventing future flares, it's important to learn the following:

- The sources of various toxins
- How to lower your exposure to toxins
- How to reverse the damaging effects of toxins on your body

This chapter will tell you which chemicals may contribute to and trigger IBD, and how to lower your toxic load from meals, beverages, and other products you use in daily life.

Let's take a closer look at 4 types of toxins that may contribute to IBD:

1. **Toxic Drugs**: antibiotics, birth control pills, hormone replacement therapy, NSAIDs (Non-Steroidal Anti-inflammatory Medication), and acne treatments

2. **Dietary Toxins**: processed foods, inflammatory foods, and tap water
3. **Environmental Toxins**: personal care products, cleaning products, plastics
4. **Toxic Emotions**: stress, anger, resentment, bitterness, helplessness

Toxic Drugs

Did you know that certain drugs can trigger the development of IBD? Studies show that drugs such as antibiotics, birth control pills, hormone replacement therapy, NSAIDs (Non-Steroidal Anti-inflammatory Medication), and acne medications can cause ulcerative colitis and Crohn's disease. Let's review these medications.[1]

Antibiotics

Antibiotics are used in treatments

Antibiotics are powerful medications that are used to treat bacterial and parasitic infections. For example, you will be prescribed antibiotics if you have sinus infection, urinary tract infection, ear infection, pneumonia, or parasitic infection such as Giardia intestinalis or Entamoeba histolytica. Antibiotics can stop the infection and save your life. However, taking antibiotics can lead to serious side effects, such as increased risk of IBD, bloody diarrhea, abdominal pain, and yeast infections.

In 2019, the CDC issued a warning on antibiotics: "Any antibiotic use carries the potential for side effects, such as diarrhea and yeast infections that naturally result from disrupting our microbiome. Some antibiotics can also lead to side effects that are severe, disabling, and even deadly."[2]

The latest study done by Harvard Medical School and Karolinska Institute in Sweden confirms that "patients treated with antibiotics three or more times had a 55% increased risk for IBD, compared to those with no previous antibiotic prescriptions".

Researchers concluded that frequent use of broad-spectrum antibiotics permanently alters gut microbiomes, promoting proliferation of fungi, particularly *Candida albicans,* which is considered a trigger for IBD. The study was published in 2020 in The Lancet Gastroenterology & Hepatology.[3, 4]

How You Ingest Antibiotics with Your Food

Even if you don't take prescription antibiotics yourself, you might unknowingly ingest antibiotics in your food - particularly meat, seafood, and dairy.

Antibiotics are routinely mixed with animal feed in order to promote quick weight gain in pigs, cows, and poultry, and to prevent disease in crowded barns, especially in the United States. Farmed fish and shellfish also have antibiotics added to their tanks to prevent disease.

"Of all antibiotics sold in the United States, approximately 80% are sold for use in animal agriculture; about 70% of these are "medically important" (i.e., from classes important to human medicine)."[5]

Europe banned antibiotic use in animal feed in 2006. Markos Kyprianou, European Commissioner for Health and Consumer Protection, said:

> *"This ban on antibiotics as growth promoters is of great importance, not only as part of the EU's food safety strategy, but also when considering public health. We need to greatly reduce the non-essential use of antibiotics if we are to effectively address the problem of micro-organisms becoming resistant to treatments that we have relied on for years. Animal feed is the first step in the food chain, and so a good place to take action in trying to meet this objective."*[6]

Unfortunately, the U.S. food industry continues to use antibiotics in animal feed.

Antibiotics foster drug-resistant "bad" bacteria

In 2010, the FDA stated:

> *"Giving animals antibiotics in order to increase food production is a threat to public health and should be stopped."*

FDA Deputy Commissioner Joshua Sharfstein, MD, said at a news conference:

> *"It's a public health issue when antibiotics important for human health are given to animals on a massive scale. Such use encourages the growth of drug-resistant bacteria that can cause hard-to-treat human disease."* [7]
>
> *"The CDC estimates that in the United States, more than two million people are sickened every year with antibiotic-resistant infections, with at least 23,000 dying as a result."* [8]

Antibiotics kill "good" bacteria

Your gut microbiome is a community of naturally occurring microbes. A healthy gut microbiome is vital; it supports the immune system and prevents disease.

The microbes we call "bad" are the ones that cause infection. And the microbes we call "good" are the ones that protect us from infection. Antibiotics kill both "bad" and "good" microbes. It can take months for "good" microbes to come back, which leaves us with a damaged microbiome that can contribute to the disease process.

Dr. Cecilla Jernberg, et al. from Karolinska Institute in Sweden, documented in her study that "healthy volunteers treated for 1 week or less with antibiotics, reported effects on their bacterial flora that persisted six months to two years after treatment, including a dramatic loss in diversity as well as in representation of specific taxa, insurgence of antibiotic resistant strains, and up-regulation of antibiotic resistance genes".[9]

So, taking antibiotics for just 7 days can negatively affect your gut flora for *up to two years*. And that's for healthy people. Imagine what antibiotics can do to people whose flora is already impaired, such as IBD patients.

Antibiotics use may be especially damaging to children

"Surveys on thousands of children have highlighted a link between the use of antibiotics during the first year of life and development of asthma by the sixth-seventh year." [9]

Antibiotic use in infants resulted in disruption of healthy intestinal flora and development of antibiotic resistant genes.[9]

Antibiotics increase probability of becoming sick with IBD

The latest study done by Harvard Medical School and Karolinska Institute in Sweden confirms that "patients treated with antibiotics three or more times had a 55% increased risk for IBD, compared to those with no previous antibiotic prescriptions".[10]

Researchers concluded that frequent use of broad-spectrum antibiotics permanently alters gut microbiome, promoting proliferation of fungi, particularly *Candida albicans,* which is considered a trigger for IBD. The study was published in 2020 in The Lancet Gastroenterology & Hepatology.[11]

Another study done in Canada shows a clear "association between the use of antibiotics and new diagnoses of Crohn's disease and ulcerative colitis". After studying 2,234 people diagnosed with IBD, researchers concluded that individuals who took numerous courses of antibiotics within a 2–5-year period had a 50% probability of becoming sick with IBD.[12]

Birth Control Pills (Oral Contraceptives) and Hormone Replacement Therapy

Do you know that birth control pills and hormone replacement therapy are linked to increased risk of IBD?

Birth Control Pills Increase Risk of IBD and GI surgery

Based on 14 studies published in 2008, it was confirmed "that current use of oral contraceptives is associated with a nearly 50% increase in risk of CD" (Crohn's disease). The longer a woman uses the birth control pill, the higher her risk of getting sick with IBD.

Why does that happen? A hypothesis is that oral estrogen in birth control pills changes the gut microbiome and increases intestinal permeability (aka leaky gut). All that contributes to the development of autoimmune disease. Furthermore, oral contraceptives may promote the increase of inflammatory cytokines (Th-1 and Th-2) that result in excessive inflammatory response and tissue damage.[13]

Harvard University gastroenterologist Dr. Hamed Khalili led a landmark study of 232,452 American women spanning over three decades, lasting from 1976 to 2008. Dr. Khalili and his associates compared the gut health of women who took birth control pills to women who never used birth control pills.

Gastroenterology journal published in 2016 summarizes Dr. Hamed Khalili study:

"Estrogen-containing oral contraceptive use has been associated with an increased risk of Crohn's disease (CD) since the 1970s". "Khalili et al report an increased risk of CD-related surgery with ≥3 years of oral combined estrogen-progestin contraceptive use after diagnosis."[14, 15]

So, this means if a woman with Crohn's disease is using estrogen-containing oral contraceptives for more than 3 years, she has an increased risk of having intestinal surgery.

Hormone Replacement Therapy increases risk of Ulcerative Colitis

According to Dr. Khalili, women on hormone replacement therapy (HRT) had a 1.7 times higher risk of ulcerative colitis, versus women who never used HRT. Estrogen use affects the colon's permeability, making it more susceptible to inflammation.[16]

NSAIDs increase risk of developing IBD

Today, more people than ever routinely take NSAIDs (nonsteroidal anti-inflammatory drugs). Aspirin and Advil are typical representatives of NSAIDs. For some people, it's habitual to pop an aspirin for a headache, or take Advil for joint pain. Most NSAIDs do not require prescription, and are casually used by people to treat headaches, menstrual cramps, fever, inflammation, injuries, muscle pain, and joint pain.

Here are some of the most common NSAIDs:

- Ibuprofen: Advil, Advil Migraine, Motrin, Midol Maximum Strength Cramp Formula
- Aspirin: Bayer Aspirin, Ecotrin, St. Joseph Aspirin, Stanback Analgesic
- Naproxen: Aleve, Naprosyn, All Day Pain Relief, Aleve Caplet, Prevacid NapraPac 375
- Diclofenac sodium: Voltaren, Solaraze

If you use NSAIDs frequently and in large doses, you might suffer from stomach pain, diarrhea, heartburn, and stomach/intestinal ulcers. These symptoms may be mild or severe, or they may be hardly detectable. In any case, NSAIDs adversely affect intestinal flora. Therefore, some individuals who frequently use NSAIDs can develop ulcerative colitis or Crohn's disease.

A study was presented at the American College of Gastroenterology (ACG) 2011 Annual Scientific Meeting. Here what it says:

1. "High doses of nonsteroidal anti-inflammatory drugs (NSAIDs), longer duration of use, or greater frequency of use are all associated with an increased risk for Crohn's disease and ulcerative colitis"
2. Also, "compared with nonusers, women who used NSAIDs for more than 15 days a month faced a greater risk for Crohn's disease and ulcerative colitis."[17]

In 2000, The American Journal of Gastroenterology published a study on the relationship between NSAIDs usage and IBD onset/exacerbation. The results of the study were shocking: "In 31% of our IBD population there was a correlation between use of NSAIDs and IBD activity." Dr. Felder and his team from the prestigious New York University School of Medicine and Lenox Hills Hospital concluded that "NSAIDs provoke disease activity in both ulcerative colitis and Crohn's disease and should be avoided in patients with a history of IBD whenever possible".[18]

Acne treatment with Isotretinoin is a risk factor for IBD

Isotretinoin is a drug used for the treatment and prevention of acne. Isotretinoin was sold under the brand name of Accutane. However, Accutane is no longer available in the U.S. Now, isotretinoin is sold under the following names: Amnesteem, Sotret, Claravis, Absorica, Myorisan, Zenatane.

One of my patients had acne; his dermatologist prescribed Accutane tablets, ingested orally. After a few months of taking Accutane, this young man began to experience severe stomach pain, diarrhea, and rectal bleeding. He was diagnosed with ulcerative colitis.

Later, he learned that oral Accutane has serious side effects, including liver damage, nausea, vomiting, bloody diarrhea, ulcerative colitis, and Crohn's disease.

Over 7000 people who took Accutane filed lawsuits against Roche (the drug maker of Accutane). While some blamed Accutane for depression, psychosis, and suicide, most of filed lawsuits were for IBD. Roche was accused of knowing that Accutane can cause serious gastrointestinal problems.[19]

One of the plaintiffs, Andrew McCarrell, claimed that after taking Accutane in 1995, he developed severe ulcerative colitis in the summer of 1996. He suffered from vomiting, diarrhea, pain, and fatigue. In December of 1996, Andrew's entire colon and rectum was surgically removed. An ileoanal pouch was installed. In the next 6 years, Andrew endured multiple surgeries and complications including pain, diarrhea, and leakage of fecal matter. In the summer of 2003, Andrew McCarrell filed a lawsuit against Roche. In 2017, a New Jersey Supreme court awarded McCarrell $25 million dollars for his pain and suffering.[20, 21]

Dietary Toxins from Gut Damaging Foods

What you eat determines whether you'll be sick or healthy. I must admit - before I got sick, I loved eating chocolate chip cookies, crunchy potato chips, and ice-cold coke with extra-cheesy pizza. I loved the taste, and I loved the convenience. Back then, I did not know that these foods are highly processed and loaded with sugar, harmful fats, and toxic chemicals.

Years went by, and I began to realize that the Standard American Diet (SAD for short - no pun intended, but it is sad indeed) is full of gut-damaging foods and ingredients. Just look at all the snacks filled with preservatives, processed meat loaded with emulsifiers, and drinks infused with artificial sugars and flavors. Over time, these toxic foods produce a negative impact on the digestive system by triggering the destruction of beneficial gut flora, damaging the gut lining, and causing inflammation.

Again, for people afflicted with IBD, these negative effects are greatly exacerbated, and are especially dangerous. You must be aware of these toxic, gut-damaging foods in order to avoid them:

- GMO Foods
- Trans fats and refined oils
- Sugar
- Artificial Colors
- Food Preservatives
- Food Additives
- Artificial Flavors
- Artificial Sweeteners
- Emulsifiers
- Citric Acid
- Beverages to Avoid
- Alcohol

Let's discuss them one by one.

GMOs

GM (genetically modified) foods, aka GMOs (genetically modified organisms) are problematic for colitis & Crohn's patients.

The Integrative Physicians Group in Scottsdale, Arizona says GMOs are a growing health risk. They note:

> *"Specifically, a higher risk for allergies, toxic intestinal bacteria, reduced immune function, and liver problems. These risks apply to everyone, but especially those with inflammatory bowel disease. For a patient with Crohn's disease or ulcerative colitis, they're devastating, making it difficult for patients to recover properly. Ultimately, GMOs create bowel hypersensitivity, increase inflammation and damage to the intestinal lining. This makes IBD and IBS cases much worse, as they contribute and, in some cases, may actually trigger these diseases."* [22]

GMOs may impair immunity and the digestive system

IBD patients, due to their damaged intestinal flora, have impaired immunity to begin with. Ingestion of GM foods can accelerate damage to an already weakened and inflamed digestive system.

GMOs may kill good bacteria

GM foods contain pesticide residue known to kill good gut bacteria, allowing bad gut bacteria to multiply rapidly. In time, you end up in a vicious cycle of dysbiosis (altered gut flora), impaired immunity, and inflammation. Therefore, IBD patients should remove GM foods from their diet to allow good bacteria to grow, and to prevent growth of bad bacteria.

GMOs may be related to food allergies that trigger flares

Food allergies/sensitivities can trigger flares in ulcerative colitis and Crohn's. Two of the most common food allergens are soy and corn - they also happen to be two of the most common GM foods.

The American Academy of Environmental Medicine (AAEM), an international association of physicians, released this statement:

"Multiple animal studies have shown that GM foods cause damage to various organ systems in the body. With this mounting evidence, it is imperative to have a moratorium [ban] on GM foods for the safety of our patients' and the public's health."[23]

The AAEM states:

- "Several animal studies indicate serious health risks associated with GM food consumption including infertility, immune dysregulation, accelerated aging, dysregulation of genes associated with cholesterol synthesis, insulin regulation, cell signaling, and protein formation, and changes in the liver, kidney, spleen and gastrointestinal system."

- "Because GM foods have not been properly tested for human consumption, and because there is ample evidence of probable harm, the AAEM asks: Physicians to educate their patients, the medical community, and the public to avoid GM foods when possible and provide educational materials concerning GM foods and health risks."
- "Physicians to consider the possible role of GM foods in the disease processes of the patients they treat and to document any changes in patient health when changing from GM food to non-GM food."[24]

How do GMOs affect humans?

A GMO (genetically modified organism) is created by scientists in a laboratory. Scientists take genes from one species and insert these genes into another species, in order to develop a new trait. Genetic modification extends even to splicing together plant, animal, bacteria, and virus genes - these trait combinations do not occur in nature.

That is how GM (genetically modified) corn was created. Scientists wanted to modify corn to be pest resistant. They took genes from Bacillus thuringiensis (Bt), a soil bacterium that produces insecticidal toxins. Then, they spliced the Bt genes into corn genes, so that the corn itself produced the insecticidal toxin, aka Bt-toxin.

When this genetically modified corn grows in a field, a bug might eat the corn. The Bt-toxin produced by the corn would then rupture the bug's stomach, killing it. You cannot wash off Bt-toxin because every plant cell in this GM corn has Bt-toxin built into its structure.

At first, scientists assumed that Bt-toxin would only destroy insects, without affecting humans.

However, according to Jeffrey Smith, GMO researcher and a consumer advocate:

"A 2011 study published in the Journal of Applied Toxicology showed that when Bt-toxin derived from Monsanto's corn was exposed to human cells, the toxin disrupts the membrane in just 24 hours, causing certain fluid to leak through the cell walls.

The authors specifically note, 'This may be due to pore formation like in insect cells.' In other words, the toxin may be creating small holes in human cells in the same manner that it kills insects.

The researchers 'documented that modified Bt-toxins [from GM plants] are not inert on human cells but can exert toxicity.'

A 2011 Canadian study conducted at Sherbrooke Hospital discovered that 93% of the pregnant women they tested had Bt-toxin from Monsanto's corn in their blood. And so did 80% of their unborn fetuses. If Bt-toxin causes allergies, then gene transfer carries serious ramifications. If Bt genes relocate to human gut bacteria, our intestinal flora may be converted into living pesticide factories, possibly producing Bt-toxin inside of us year after year."[25]

How did these women end up having so much Bt-toxin in their blood? We can assume they were consuming food and drinks made from GMOs. GM corn is extremely common - it's found in cereal, tacos, drinks with high fructose corn syrup, and other processed foods.

If so much Bt-toxin is found inside living humans, what effect could that have on their digestive systems? Turns out, there is strong scientific evidence that GM foods can cause severe stomach inflammation, cancer, and premature death in animals. Here are the studies.

Study #1: GMO causes cancer and premature death in rats

Interestingly, biotech companies often use only short (90 day) studies on GM foods and Roundup. However, long-term studies deliver more insight on long-term effects.

Here is the only long-term study (2 years) on both GMO corn and Roundup, a pesticide used in growing GMO corn. The study was published by Seralini et al. The researchers demonstrated that rats eating GM corn suffered liver and kidney damage, grew huge cancerous tumors, and died prematurely.

Here is a short summary of the study:

"Séralini's is the first long-term peer-reviewed toxicity study on the health impacts of GM NK603 maize and the commercial herbicide formulation it is engineered to be grown with. GM food crops are authorized on the basis of short (a maximum of 90 days) feeding studies, usually carried out in rats. Long-term studies are not required by regulators anywhere in the world. But in Séralini's study the first large tumours were only seen four months into the trial in the case of males and seven months in the case of females. Most tumours were only detected after 18 months. This shows that the 90-day tests routinely done on GM crops are not long enough to detect serious health effects that take time to develop, such as cancer and organ damage. Ninety days in a rat is equivalent to only 7–9 years in human terms – yet human beings could eat GM food and residues of Roundup over a lifetime."[26]

Study #2: GMO feed causes severe stomach inflammation in pigs

Dr. Judy Carman at Flinders University in Adelaide, Australia, demonstrated a strong connection between animals ingesting GMO feed and severe damage to their digestive systems. The 6-month study used 168 pigs: one group of pigs was fed GMO corn and soy, and the other group was fed non-GMO corn and soy.

Dr. Carman found,

> *"GM-fed pigs showed severe stomach inflammation at a rate of 2.6 times that of non-GM-fed pigs." The study added: "Humans have a similar gastrointestinal tract to pigs, and these GM crops are widely consumed by people, particularly in the USA." The author emphasizes that long-term animal feeding studies with GM crops should be done prior to planting GM foods used for human consumption.*[27]

What foods contain GMOs?

American people consume GMO-containing foods every day without even knowing it. Over 70% of foods in your local supermarket contain GM ingredients, including genetically modified corn, soy, canola, and sugar beets. These GM foods are used to create products such as breakfast cereals, corn chips, potato chips, soft drinks, sweetened yogurt, infant formula, salad dressings, bread, cereal, hamburgers, mayonnaise, veggie burgers, meat substitutes, soy cheese, tomato sauce, crackers, cookies, chocolate, candy, fried food, protein powder, baking powder, alcohol, vanilla, sugar, peanut butter, ice cream, frozen yogurt, tofu, tamari, and soy sauce. Quite a list.

IBD patients should avoid GM foods

Until we get to see long-term clinical studies on humans and GM food safety, it makes sense for people with ulcerative colitis and Crohn's disease to avoid GM foods. Since GM foods are not labeled in the U.S., the only way you can avoid GM foods is to buy whole, USDA-certified, 100% organic foods.

How to avoid GMOs

1. **Become an educated consumer.**

   Purchase organic or non-GMO certified foods. Check out http://knowyourgut.com/resources for links to Non-GMO Shopping Guides that can help you identify brands and food products that are GM-free.

   If you're curious to see which foods are currently approved to be genetically modified (GM), you can view the list, at the International Service for the Acquisition of Agri-biotech Applications (ISAAA) GM approval database. You'll find out that a wide range of genetically modified grains, vegetables, fruits, seeds, nuts, and spices are on the market.

2. **Find organically grown food at your local farmer's market.**

   I buy from local farmers who grow their produce organically, even if they don't have organic certification. Maintaining organic certification can be expensive for small farms. Talk to sellers at the farmer's market about where they get their produce and ask which pesticides they use.

   Be aware that some people simply buy produce wholesale and resell it to you. I try not to buy from these stands - most of the time, their produce is not organic. Also, I try to support local farms and farmers; they are intimately involved in the process of growing food for their families and their customers, and it shows.

   Check out http://knowyourgut.com/resources for links to local farmers markets and community-supported agriculture:

3. **Plant your own garden.**

   Another way to secure quality food is to grow your own organic herbs and produce. It is fun and rewarding, plus it will ensure you have the best food for your gut. You will know exactly how your fruits and vegetables are grown. Also, having a garden can save a ton of money on your grocery bill.

Trans fats and Refined Oils

Trans fats and refined oils are another common item to look out for in your food. Let's learn about them.

What are trans fats?

Trans fats are created by adding hydrogen to liquid oils. This creates solid fat, like margarine. You can identify trans fats by reading ingredient labels. Trans fats are listed on labels as "hydrogenated fats".

What's so bad about trans fats?

A study of 170,805 women published in the journal Gut shows that eating lots of trans fats may increase risk of ulcerative colitis, whereas consuming lots of long-chain n-3 PUFA, found in oily fish or fish oil may decrease risk of ulcerative colitis.[28]

So, if you already have colitis and Crohn's, stay away from foods that are high in trans fats such as French fries, coffee creamer, frozen pizza, frozen pies, crackers, cookies, cakes, some margarines, vegetable shortenings, and any food that has hydrogenated vegetable oil on its ingredient list.

What are refined oils?

Refined oils are created using harmful chemicals. Their original source is corn, soybeans, rapeseeds, cottonseed, safflower seeds, or peanuts. The refined oil extraction process uses solvents and other chemicals. First, the oilseeds or nuts are heated to a high temperature to extract the oil. After extraction is completed, the solvent (n-hexane) is added to extract additional oil. Then, the oil is refined, bleached, and deodorized to remove odor, bitterness, and color. The end product is refined oil that contains trans fats, chemical residues, and additives; that doesn't sound like real food to me.

What is so bad about refined oils?

Refined vegetable oils are high in omega-6 fatty acids that promote inflammation and increase disease risk. Scientists from Harvard Medical School conducted a study where they fed mice a diet high in omega-6 fatty acids. As a result of this diet, mice experienced systemic inflammation and endotoxemia (changes in the permeability of the intestinal flora).[29]

Our bodies need fats like omega-6 and omega 3, because we cannot synthesize them. So, we must get these fats from food. To maintain good health, we should eat a 1:1 ratio of omega-6 to omega-3 fats. The modern

Western diet has an excess of unhealthy omega-6 fats, and a lack of omega-3 fats. In the modern Western diet, healthy animal fats are often substituted with highly processed and toxic vegetable oils, margarines, and other processed foods. That is why the current ratio of omega-6 to omega-3 fats in today's Western diet is extremely imbalanced, with an average ratio of 16:1.[30]

Refined oils contribute to the development of chronic, degenerative, inflammatory diseases such as fatty liver, cardiovascular problems, rheumatoid arthritis, and IBD.

I suggest avoiding refined vegetable oils such as soybean, canola, corn, grapeseed, sunflower, cottonseed, peanut oil, as well as processed foods containing them.

If you are serious about your recovery, ditch margarines, mayonnaise, salad dressings, and any food containing refined oils.

However, keep in mind that not all omega-6 fats are harmful. If you choose whole foods like walnuts, pumpkin seed, sunflower seeds, and avocados, you will get healthy, naturally occurring omega-6 fatty acids.

In this program, I recommend using the following oils:

1. Organic, extra virgin cold pressed olive oil. This oil is high in antioxidants and healthy monounsaturated fatty acids. Multiple studies found that people living in regions with high consumption of olive oil had a lower risk of breast cancer and colon cancer. This oil is a staple in my kitchen.
2. Organic, cold pressed coconut oil. This oil is high in medium chain triglycerides (MCT), which is a specific type of acid which is super easy to digest and absorb, which is crucial, especially at the time of IBD flare. I also like coconut oil because it can improve the digestion of fat-soluble vitamins (A, D, E and K).

Sugar

Some people label sugar as "white death". I don't want to say that sugar can kill you - it might be alright in small amounts for healthy people. I do know that eating too much of it, especially if you have IBD, can lead to inflammation, leaky gut, and intestinal tissue damage in addition to diabetes, heart disease, obesity, and tooth decay.

It's a fact: "the people of the US consume more sugar than any other country in the world. On average, Americans consume 126.4 grams of sugar daily. That represents ¼ of a pound and more than 10 times the lowest recommendation!"[31]

The average American consumes about 152 pounds of sugar a year. This is equal to 12 pounds, or 24 cups of sugar consumed in just one month! Just compare it to two hundred years ago, when the average American ate just 2 pounds a year.[32]

How Added Sugar Affects Your Gut

A diet high in sugar is linked to an increased risk of inflammation and death

American Journal of Clinical Nutrition published a study in 2010, which included analysis of a food-frequency questionnaire for 1490 women and 1245 men. "Over a 13-year period, 84 women and 86 men died of inflammatory diseases."

High intake of food high in refined sugars and low intake of vegetables (excluding potatoes) was linked to an increased risk of inflammation and death.[33]

A diet high in sugar increases risk of ulcerative colitis and Crohn's disease.

A large study on "the dietary patterns and risk of inflammatory bowel disease (IBD)" of people living in Europe. Multiple scientists from

France, Germany, Italy, Denmark, the Netherlands, Sweden, & the UK "found that sugar and soft drinks are associated with increased risk of ulcerative colitis (UC)."

Furthermore, "multiple studies during the 1970s and 1990s had well documented an association between sugar consumption and CD".[34]

So, what happens when we eat too much sugar?

According to mice study done at the University of Alberta, Canada, sugar dramatically changes gut bacteria and "feeds bad microbes, such as E. coli, that are associated with inflammation and a defective immune response."

According to Karen Madsen, that led this study and "who specializes in diet and its effects on inflammatory bowel disease, said:

> *"It has been previously shown that the type of diet that you are on can change your susceptibility to disease. We wanted to know how long it takes before a change in diet translates into an impact on health. In the case of sugar and colitis, it only took two days, which was really surprising to us. We didn't think it would happen so quickly." "The results echo what many patients with colitis have been saying for a long time: small changes in their diet can make their symptoms flare up."*

Also, this study also showed that mice eating a high-sugar diet experienced intestinal lining damage and impaired immune response.[35]

Sugar quality

You should also consider the quality of sugar you are eating.

Today, about 98% of sugar beets in the U.S. are grown as GM (genetically modified) beets. These GMO beets are used to produce 4.5 million tons of sugar in the United States.[36]

This GM sugar is added to foods that people eat daily, such as sweetened yogurt, cereals, crackers, soups, canned foods, peanut butter, candies, cakes, cookies, pastries, ice-cream, flavored oats, granola bars, protein bars, pasta sauces, salad dressings, sport drinks, energy drinks, and juice drinks.

So, what's the big deal with GMO sugar? Well, it often contains glyphosate residue. Glyphosate is a weed killer that was classified by the World Health Organization (WHO) as "probably carcinogenic in humans." Moreover, when you consume glyphosate, it acts as an antibiotic, which kills beneficial intestinal flora and promotes the rapid growth of pathogens in your gut.

Bottom Line: If you are serious about healing your gut, remove all genetically modified sugar from your diet for good.

Furthermore, you can reduce inflammation in your body and heal leaky gut by eliminating most of the added sugar and processed carbs from your diet. The following inflammation-promoting foods should be off your menu: soda, white bread, white pasta, and any foods containing sucrose, fructose, glucose, high-fructose corn syrup, maltose, and dextrose.

Artificial Sweeteners

If you think that sugar is bad, and that artificial sweeteners are good, you must reconsider!

Artificial sweeteners can do the following:

- Double the risk for Crohn's disease
- Destroy your beneficial gut flora
- Cause abdominal, joint pain, nausea/vomiting, allergic reactions, type 2 diabetes, obesity, and migraine headaches

Artificial sweeteners (aka fake sugar, sugar-free, or zero calorie sweetener) can include aspartame, Splenda (sucralose), saccharin, and acesulfame potassium.

Artificial sweeteners can be found in:

- meal replacement drinks, diet soda, sport drinks, fruit juice
- canned fruit, dried fruit, yogurt, nutrition bars, shake mixes, jams
- instant flavored oatmeal, cereal, bread, English muffins
- gelatin desserts, milk drinks, instant tea and coffees, hot cocoa, wine coolers

These foods are often labeled as "sugar-free", "low-sugar", or "light".

Artificial sweetener can double your risk for IBD

A recent study published in 2018 in Inflammatory Bowel Disease Journal showed that the artificial sweetener sucralose (aka Splenda) increased intestinal inflammation when given to mice with Crohn's-like disease. This study revealed that artificial sweeteners promote intestinal dysbiosis, increase inflammation, and worsen symptoms in Crohn's Disease. This is because sucralose reduces the number of gut beneficial bacteria. With less beneficial bacteria in your gut, pathogens tend to multiply quickly.[37]

Fake sugars can destroy your beneficial gut microflora

According to a 2008 animal study published in the Journal of Toxicology and Environmental Health, artificial sweeteners can increase the pH level in the intestines of male rats and reduce the number of beneficial bacteria by a whopping 50%. So, the truth is out: Splenda can have adverse effects on beneficial gut microflora.[38]

Dr. Xiaofa Qin from the Department of Surgery in New Jersey Medical School states:

> *"a series of findings made me suspect that saccharin may be a key causative factor for IBD, through its inhibition on gut bacteria and the resultant impaired inactivation of digestive proteases and over digestion of the mucus layer and gut barrier (the Bacteria-Protease-Mucus-Barrier hypothesis)."*

> *"Recently I further found evidence suggesting sucralose may be also linked to IBD through a similar mechanism as saccharin and have contributed to the recent worldwide increase of IBD."*

Dr. Qin's decades-long research shows ample evidence that artificial sweeteners such as sucralose and saccharin are directly connected to development of IBD. [39]

The Bottom Line: Now you know that artificial sweeteners radically change your microbiome and are a hidden trigger for IBD. Make an effort to read ingredient list to avoid all artificial sweeteners. A diet full of artificial sugars is detrimental to your health, especially to your gut.

The Bitter Truth about Stevia

You would be shocked to know that I currently recommend my patients *to stay away from stevia*! I know it sounds confusing, especially when stevia is heavily marketed as a healthy, natural sweetener. But there is NOTHING natural about stevia!

Let me explain…

Years ago, I bought organic stevia powder, which I used to prepare homemade cherry jello. For breakfast, I ate 2 cups of this jello on an empty stomach. Pretty soon, I became bloated, gassy, and had diarrhea. I could not believe it! I thought organic stevia powder was safe. I was so wrong! So, I started to investigate how so-called "natural" stevia sweeteners are made. Here is what I learned.

In nature, stevia plants have leaves that are naturally sweet. To transform green leaves into white powder or liquid sweetener takes a lot of processing and toxic chemicals. The final product is far removed from the natural stevia leaves. Stevia liquid and powder that is sold in groceries and health food stores is a highly processed, toxic product mixed with sugar alcohols and maltodextrin (made from GMO corn) to create a sweet taste.

It turns out that the sugar alcohols (erythritol and sorbitol) that are part of stevia products are known to cause gas, bloating, diarrhea, and even irritable bowel syndrome, especially in large doses. Even healthy adults and children can get affected by sugar alcohols.[40]

Stevia Can Kill Beneficial Bacteria in Your Gut

Scientists from the Institute of Microbiology and Biotechnology from the University of Latvia demonstrated that stevia sweetener suppresses the growth of six different strains of probiotic bacteria (Lactobacillus reuteri) that reside in the human gut. This allows harmful bacteria to grow, causing dysbiosis (altered gut flora).[41]

So, it turns out stevia not only causes digestive distress - it can also disturb your microflora.

Attention IBD people: do you really need more abdominal pain and diarrhea after your meals like I experienced after using stevia?

The Bottom Line: Stevia powder or drops are not a healthy option for your gut. Stevia is just another fake sugar. Instead of stevia, you can use *small amounts* of natural sweeteners such as fresh and dried fruits, raw, unfiltered honey, and maple syrup. These are real sweeteners created by mother nature; they taste heavenly and are so much better for you than artificial sweeteners.

Artificial Food Coloring

Artificial food colors are chemicals used in the food industry to make food look more appetizing by enhancing or changing its color. You can find food dyes in products like sport drinks, soda, jello, fruit roll ups, cereal bars, kid's frozen meals, sausages, boxed mac & cheese, candies, lollipops, ice cream, sorbet, cereals, mustard, ketchup, and many other foods.

So, what's the big deal about artificial food dyes?

"Food dyes used in everything from M&Ms to Manischewitz Matzo Balls to Kraft salad dressing pose risks of cancer, hyperactivity in children, and allergies, and should be banned" according to the Center for Science in the Public Interest (CSPI).[42]

The three most popular dyes (Red 3, Red 40, & Yellow 5) are known carcinogens. Nevertheless, food manufacturers in the U.S. are adding close to 15 million pounds of artificial coloring to our foods.

"CSPI urged the FDA to ban all dyes because the scientific studies do not provide convincing evidence of safety but do provide significant evidence of harm."[42]

How Artificial Colors Contribute to Gut Inflammation

A recent study by Aristo Vojdani, PhD reveals how artificial food dyes may contribute to inflammation and leaky gut.

"Artificial food dyes are made from petroleum and have been approved by the U.S. Food and Drug Administration (FDA) for the enhancement of the color of processed foods. They are widely used in the food and pharmaceutical industries to increase the appeal and acceptability of their products."

Dr. Vojdani explains:

> *"During the past 50 years, the amount of synthetic dye used in foods has increased by 500%. The consumption of synthetic food colors, and their ability to bind with body proteins, can have significant immunological consequences. This consumption can activate the inflammatory cascade, can result in the induction of intestinal permeability to large antigenic molecules, and could lead to cross-reactivities, autoimmunities, and even neurobehavioral disorders."*

> *"More shocking is the legal number of artificial colorants allowed by the FDA in the foods, drugs, and cosmetics that we consume and use every day. The consuming public is largely unaware of the perilous truth behind the deceptive allure of artificial color."*[43]

In some European countries food coloring is banned. For example, Blue 1 is banned in France, Finland, and Norway. Yellow 5 is banned in Austria and Norway. And the rest of the European Union requires warning labels on foods containing artificial colors. This warning states that this dye "may have an adverse effect on activity and attention in children."

Sadly, food manufacturers in the U.S. are not required to have this type of warning on food containing artificial dyes. So, most consumers are not aware that they are eating these chemicals, unless they read the ingredients on the label.

Here is a list of artificial colors used in foods, drinks, drugs and supplements:

- Green Dye 3 (Fast Green)
- Blue Dye 1 (Brilliant blue) and 2 (Indigo Carmine)
- Red Dye 2 (Citrus red), Green 3 (Erythrosine) and 40 (Allura Red)
- Yellow Dye 5 (Tartrazine) and 6 (Sunset Yellow)
- Caramel coloring (often made with toxic ammonia)

The Bottom Line: By now, you have learned enough about artificial and natural dyes, so you can make healthy choices while grocery shopping. Next time you prepare for a birthday party, ditch the cakes that are colored in a rainbow of synthetic dyes and overloaded with GM sugar.

Instead, prepare a homemade, delicious dessert like dark chocolate-dipped strawberries, fruit cake, or real pumpkin cupcakes bursting with flavor and healthy ingredients like almond flour, gluten-free organic flour, nuts, raisins, dates, etc.

Artificial Flavors

Food manufacturers use hundreds of artificial flavors in order to create a certain, addictive taste. These artificial flavors were created to resemble flavors of real foods: chocolate, apple, caramel, cherry, grape, banana, orange, blueberry, strawberry, vanilla, and so on.

So, what are artificial flavors?

Artificial flavors include more than 100 chemicals that are made from petroleum, solvents, and emulsifiers. Artificial flavors may cause gut irritation, indigestion, vitamin deficiency, fatigue, genetic defects, and even cancer.

According to the Environmental Working Group:

"When foods are pasteurized for safety, many of the volatile chemicals evaporate or degrade. To make a product like orange juice taste fresh after pasteurization, these chemicals have to be restored. They dupe your taste buds and smell receptors into believing you are drinking fresh orange juice when it really may be rather old."[44]

If you see "natural flavors" in the ingredient list for your orange juice, you might be consuming these deceptive chemicals.

The Bottom Line: Do you want blueberry flavor? Eat a blueberry. Do you want chocolate flavor? Eat a piece of chocolate. You know what I mean. Don't just walk - run away from foods with artificial flavors, and choose whole, real foods instead.

Food Preservatives

Food preservation has been used by humans for centuries to extend food's shelf life, reduce spoilage, and prevent discoloration and growth of mold, yeast, and bacteria. Preservatives can be natural (such as salt, sugar, vinegar) or artificial.

There are 3 types of artificial preservatives used in food today:

- **Antioxidants** - inhibit oxidation of stored foods
- **Antimicrobial agents** - kill mold, bacteria, insects
- **Chelating agents** - bind metals during food product manufacturing

The modern food supply is flooded with artificial preservatives. Over time, these chemicals can accumulate in the body, causing serious health problems such as allergies, asthma, digestive/endocrine problems, brain damage, and cancer.

Antioxidants: Sulfites, BHA, BHT, Parabens

Sulfites (sodium/potassium sulfite, sulphur dioxide, bisulfites)

Sulfites are added to suppress the growth of bacteria in many foods: wine, beer, dried fruits, fruit juice, fruit bars, cider, gravies, sauces, jam, jellies, gelatin, bread, biscuits, pie and pizza dough, sausages, cold cuts, pickles, sauerkraut, pickles onions, etc. Sulfites are also used extensively in many cosmetics: moisturizers, facial cleansers, body washes, perfumes, tanning lotions, blush, hair colorants, and hair bleach. Consuming foods and drinks with this preservative can trigger a whole range of adverse reactions in sensitive individuals - from dermatitis, abdominal pain, and diarrhea to life-threatening anaphylactic shock.[45]

Butylated Hydroxyanisole (BHA) & Butylated Hydroxytoluene (BHT)

These preservatives are added to cereal, instant mashed potatoes, potato chips, beer, butter, nut mixed, chewing gum, snack foods, cereals, and fast foods. Both preservatives have been classified as "generally recognized to be safe" - but research on the safety of these chemicals has been done in animals and test tubes, not in people. By contrast, the state of California has listed BHA as a known carcinogen since the 1990s. BHT disrupts the endocrine system and has been linked to an increased risk of cancer in animals as well.[46]

Parabens (propylparaben, ethylparaben, methylparaben, butylparaben)

According to the CDC (Center for Disease Control and Prevention),

> *"parabens are man-made chemicals often used in small amounts as preservatives in cosmetics, pharmaceuticals, foods and beverages. People can be exposed to parabens through touching, swallowing, or eating products that contain parabens. Many products, such as makeup, moisturizers, hair-care products, and shaving creams, contain parabens. Parabens in these products are absorbed through the skin. Parabens also can enter the body when pharmaceuticals, foods, and drinks containing parabens are swallowed or eaten."*[47]

Parabens have been linked to breast cancer (in humans) and decreased sperm count (in animals). In 2006, propyl paraben preservative was banned by the European Union. Yet, the American population suffers from serious exposure to parabens. It was reported that 92.7% of Americans had propyl paraben present in their urine.[48]

Antimicrobial agents

Benzoates (Sodium Benzoate and Potassium Benzoate)

These preservatives are used as preservatives and flavoring agents. They're added to fruit juices, sodas, tea, coffee, salad dressings, jams, pickled foods, cranberry cocktails, and wine to prevent the growth of bacteria and mold.

Sodium benzoate and potassium benzoate can form benzene. The International Agency for Research on Cancer (the IARC) recognizes benzene as carcinogenic to humans.[49]

Sodium benzoate is known as E211, and potassium benzoate is known as E212.

Sodium Nitrite and Sodium Nitrate

These preservatives are added to lunch meats, bacon, hot dogs, and ham to prevent bacterial growth and prevent these processed meat products from turning brown. When we eat these processed meats, nitrite converts into nitrous acid, which is suspected to be carcinogenic. A study completed at the University of Hawaii demonstrated that people who ate the most processed meat had a 67% increase in pancreatic cancer.[50]

Sorbates (sodium sorbate, potassium sorbate)

Sorbates are added to yogurt, cheese, dried fruit, olives, pickles, soups, prepared salads, salad dressings, jam/preserves, wine, beer, soft drinks, and baked goods. Sorbic acid prevents growth of mold and fungi. Possible side effects of sorbic acid include nausea, vomiting, stomach cramps, diarrhea, and redness of skin.

Chelating agents

EDTA (Ethylenediaminetetraacetic acid)

EDTA is added to many processed foods to keep their flavor and color. Here is the list of foods that may have added EDTA: canned foods, salad dressings, sauces, mayonnaise, sodas, and pickled foods.

Although EDTA is considered safe when used in small amounts as a preservative, if you add up all foods that might have EDTA as a preservative, it might be more than you bargained for.

According to WebMD: "EDTA can cause abdominal cramps, nausea, vomiting, diarrhea, headache, low blood pressure, skin problems, and fever."[51]

Citric Acid

Modern citric acid is a common food additive which is added to many foods today as a flavoring agent and a preservative. Do not confuse synthetic citric acid with natural citric acid found in citrus fruit (e.g., lemons, limes, oranges, grapefruit, tangelos, clementines, and kumquat). When you see "citric acid" on food labels, think of black mold, which is neither natural, nor derived from citrus.

Modern Citric Acid is Made from Black Mold and Can Cause Diarrhea

Today, citric acid is synthesized from Aspergillus Niger, a black mold and common food contaminant. It's used in manufacturing citric acid because it's much cheaper than making citric acid from citrus. First, the manufacturers start with sucrose or glucose made from GMO corn starch. Then, they introduce the black mold. The black mold converts sugars into a citric acid solution. According to the University of Michigan Medicine, modern citric acid has serious side effects such as ongoing diarrhea, severe stomach pain, bloody stool, numbness, mood changes, and seizures.[52]

The U.S. National Organic Program allows foods labeled organic to contain up to 5% non-organic ingredients. That is why you might see non-organic citric acid added to organic foods.

Did you know that citric acid is commonly added to the following foods?

- Baby food
- Cheese
- Caramel candies
- Canned foods and sauces
- Dips, spreads, and hummus
- Frozen fish, canned fish, and shellfish
- Processed sweets, baked goods, breads
- Pre-cut and packaged vegetables and fruits

Did you know that citric acid is added to the following medications?

- Cabergoline
- Diurex
- Effervescent potassium
- Mefenamic acid
- Parcopa
- Simvastatin
- Tri-buffered aspirin
- Unisom Sleep Melts
- Zolpidem Tartrate

Citric Acid in Baby Food can cause Acid Reflux in Babies

Parents beware! Citric acid is often added to commercial baby food. Now you know why some babies experience acid reflux and digestive symptoms after eating store-bought baby foods.

Citric Acid in Metamucil

Metamucil is a popular brand of fiber supplements, recommended by doctors to adults and children for constipation relief. But here is the deal: while natural psyllium husk is the main ingredient in Metamucil, citric acid is added as preservative, along with other gut-disturbing ingredients, such as sugar (sucrose), and a coloring agent (FD&C Yellow No. 6) that gives Metamucil its bright orange color.

The Bottom Line: Read food and supplements labels and avoid citric acid at all costs; it can cause serious digestive problems. If you have a baby, it would be ideal to prepare homemade food for your little one. It's so much better for your child than anything you can buy packaged at the store. Also, if your medications contain citric acid, ask your doctor for a citric acid-free substitute.

Artificial preservatives have no place in your gut-healing diet. Stick to fresh fruits, vegetables, legumes, and nuts. Stay away from packaged foods. Employ healthy food preservation methods at home: freezing, dehydration, canning, fermentation, and pickling of whole, organic foods.

Food Additives

The U.S. allows food additives that are banned in Europe, specifically potassium bromate and azodicarbonamide (also known as ACA).

Potassium bromate is often added to flour, as an additive to help bread rise and to make bread whiter and fluffier. You can find bromated, bleached, refined flour in packaged bread, breadcrumbs, bagel chips, and hamburger/hot dog buns. Bromated flour is linked to GI distress, thyroid and kidney cancer, and it's banned in The European Union, Brazil, and China - however, it's still used in the U.S.

Azodicarbonamide (ADA) is another dangerous chemical. It is used as a "foaming agent" to create gas bubbles in vinyl plastics. It is also used as a dough conditioner and to whiten dough in baked goods. However, when the final product is baked, ADA breaks down into 2 chemicals: urethane and semi carbazide. The U.S. Department of Health and Human Services states that urethane is "reasonably anticipated to be a human carcinogen."[53]

So, when you bite into name-brand breadsticks made from a tube of dough, fast food croissants, buns, or sourdough bread, you could be eating ADA as part of your meal. According to EWG (Environmental Working Group) ADA "is listed as an ingredient on the labels of many well-known brands of bread, croutons, pre-made sandwiches and snacks, including Ball Park, Butternut, Country Hearth, Fleischman's, Food Club, Harvest Pride, Healthy Life, Jimmy Dean, Joseph Campione, Kroger, Little Debbie, Mariano's, Marie Callender's, Martin's, Mother's, Pillsbury, Roman Meal, Sara Lee, Schmidt, Shoprite, Safeway, Smucker's, Sunbeam, Turano, Tyson, Village Hearth and Wonder". ADA "is not approved for use in either Australia or the European Union."[54]

Gum Additives can trigger intestinal ulcers

Strong acids, formaldehyde, and chlorine bleach are used to manufacture gum additives. Gum additives are used as thickening, emulsifying agents. Examples include carrageenan, xanthan gum, guar gum, and locust bean gum. These additives add texture and increase viscosity in foods such as yogurt, sorbets, ice cream, puddings, chocolates, mayonnaise, deli meats, frozen foods, protein powders, and non-dairy beverages like soymilk, almond milk, coconut, or hazelnut milk. Added gums in foods create a smooth and thick consistency, but can trigger severe bloating, abdominal pain, and diarrhea in people with IBD.

Carrageenan

What is carrageenan?

Carrageenan is a gum extracted from red seaweed. Many manufacturers use it as a thickener. It's very common and you can find it in puddings, jams, milkshakes, sauces, ice cream, cottage cheese, yogurt, baked goods, and soy milk. Quite a list, isn't it?

What's so bad about carrageenan?

Carrageenan can induce bloody diarrhea and intestinal ulcers leading to inflammatory diseases like colitis. Scientists found that giving mice drinking water with a 10% carrageenan solution caused colitis within just 10 days.[55]

In an unrelated study by Dr. Marcus and Dr. Watt, "a 5% carrageenan solution was given to guinea pigs in their drinking water from 20 to 45 days." After 2 weeks, all animals had weight loss, and after 30 days all the animals in the experimental group had blood in their feces and most had ulcers in their colon. The clinical and pathological features bear a close resemblance to human ulcerative colitis.[56]

How are these Animal Studies Related to Humans?

In both studies, carrageenan upset the natural bacteria balance of the intestines. A specific strain, Bacteroides vulgatus, was linked to ulcers in the animals. Interestingly, high numbers of the same bacteria have been found in humans who have ulcers – specifically, in the stool cultures of UC patients. So, if this bacterium is linked to ulcers in humans and animals, and carrageenan is linked to this bacterium, then it would make sense to avoid carrageenan. Until research on humans proves carrageenan is safe, patients with colitis and Crohn's should avoid foods containing carrageenan.

Xanthan Gum, Guar Gum, Locust Bean Gum

Besides carrageenan, there are other gums such as xanthan gum, guar gum, and locust bean gum (a.k.a. carob bean gum). Even a small amount of food containing these gums can trigger severe bloating, abdominal pain, and diarrhea in a person with colitis or Crohn's.

IBD patients have these reactions because there is nothing "natural" in these gums. For instance, xanthan gum is made by fermenting corn sugar with a bacteria, Xanthomonas campestris. This is the same bacteria that creates black spots on broccoli and cauliflower. The result of this fermentation is a slimy goo that is then dried up and ground into a fine white powder. Besides being an intestinal irritant - this is just plain unappetizing.

Xanthan Gum can be deadly for infants

According to Natural Health Journals: "for babies, xanthan gum should generally be avoided. In 2011, the Food and Drug Administration warned parents and caregivers of babies not to give their infants a xanthan gum-based product called SimplyThick. This powder was commonly used in hospitals to thicken breast milk or formula for infants with swallowing difficulties or to prevent spit-ups (often, in premature newborns). However, the practice was linked to necrotizing enterocolitis (NEC), a condition in which intestinal tissue becomes inflamed and dies. Of 22 babies identified as having developed NEC after being given SimplyThick, 7 died and 14 required surgeries". (Source: "Warning Too Late for Some Babies," The New York Times, Feb. 4, 2013.)[57, 58]

The Bottom Line: Pay attention and read labels! Even products that are labeled "organic", "natural", and "gluten-free" may contain one or more types of these gut-irritating gums. So, every time you buy plant milks (like soy, almond, coconut), salad dressings, protein powders/drinks, or gluten-free foods, read the label carefully! I have seen many patients suffer severe digestive reactions after consuming even small amounts of food or beverage containing gums. Do yourself a favor and avoid all products containing gums!

Emulsifiers

What are Emulsifiers?

Emulsifiers are synthetic additives used extensively in food manufacturing to improve texture and extend shelf life of baked goods, bread, margarine, ice cream, and many other processed foods. Emulsifiers prevent separation of oil and water in mayonnaise, salad dressing, and sauces. Emulsifiers help products retain a smooth and creamy texture. Who wants to bother making homemade salad dressing or sauce when you can buy one ready-to-use at the store, right?

Emulsifiers are also used in the pharmaceutical industry for better consistency in gel capsules, and in liquid medication to keep it suspended in fluid.

Polysorbate 80 and Carboxymethylcellulose lead to Inflammation

Sadly, all this texture modification and convenience comes at a price. A recent study suggests that emulsifiers alter gut flora and can activate intestinal inflammation. These symptoms are associated with ulcerative colitis and Crohn's disease.

Scientists at Georgia State University analyzed the effect of two synthetic emulsifiers, polysorbate 80 and carboxymethylcellulose (CMC), on the digestive health of mice.

These emulsifiers were added to water and given to the mice. After 12 weeks, the mice with predisposition to IBD experienced destruction to the integrity of their gut mucosal lining, intestinal inflammation, which resulted in development of "robust" colitis.[59]

Researchers stated that the incidence of inflammatory bowel disease started rising in the 20th century - around the time food manufacturers began adding emulsifiers to foods. Moreover, co-author Andrew Gewirtz, PhD. says, "We suspect some emulsifiers act like detergents, upsetting the friendly bacteria in the microbiota, which triggers low-grade inflammation and causes excess eating".

"A follow-up study by Gewirtz, a professor of biomedical sciences at Georgia State University, and his colleagues, published in Cancer Research, suggested the changes in gut bacteria from emulsifiers could trigger bowel cancer."

The FDA has labeled emulsifiers "generally recognized as safe" (GRAS), a category for food additives that do not have evidence of toxicity upon their ingestion.

"The FDA's process, they added, is not designed to detect the effects of daily consumption of an additive on such subtle measures as inflammation and microbiotic diversity."[60]

The Bottom Line: If eating synthetic emulsifiers worries you, make your own salad dressings, and avoid eating baked goods, ice cream, chocolate, or mayonnaise with added emulsifiers. Full disclosure: I avoid eating basically anything pre-made or instant that can contain emulsifiers and other harmful additives. If you want to build a strong gut, minimize your intake of any processed food.

Water Quality and Your Health

Dangerous, Toxic Chemicals in Your Tap Water

If you want to get well, you MUST consider the quality of the water you drink. We assume that the water running from our faucets is clean water. After all, clean water is a basic necessity of life. We need water to take a shower, cook food, make tea and coffee, and we drink water for hydration many times a day.

Unfortunately, our water supply is poisoned with heavy metals, disinfection byproducts, petrochemicals, fluoride, and radioactive compounds. Often, these contaminants are tasteless and invisible, with a tendency to accumulate in our bodies and cause disease.

Case in Point: a study done by the Environmental Working Group examined tap water quality in 50 states for 48,363 communities of residential water systems. These systems are in use by about 85% of U.S. homes. They found that toxic chemicals found in U.S. drinking water could be the cause of more than *100,000 cancer cases.*[61]

Over 200 Unregulated, Toxic Chemicals Found in Your Water

The EPA (Environmental Protection Agency) conducted a 3-year study on tap water in 45 states. They found that tap water contained 202 unregulated chemicals, including pharmaceuticals, weed killers, and industrial solvents. EPA tap water standards have a maximum legal limit for only 114 of these pollutants; the other 88 have no federal safety standards. The EPA does not regulate or test for radioactive substances, pesticides, and pharmaceutical residues.[62]

Fluoride in Your Water can Harm Your Brain, Bones, and Gut

Water fluoridation is promoted in the U.S. as a safe and proven way to decrease tooth decay. That is why fluoride is added to drinking water in most of the U.S.

However, the type of fluoride (fluorosilicic acid) that is added to municipal water in the U.S. is quite toxic. This type of fluoride is not natural. It's synthesized artificially and is used not only for water fluoridation, but also as insecticide and poison for rodents.

Scientific research shows that, long-term, drinking water which has been treated with industrial fluoride can cause bone fractures in the elderly. Also, fluoride is a neurotoxin. It's linked to reduced IQ and ADHD (attention deficit hyperactivity disorder) in children.

Moreover, industrial fluoride can trigger GI discomfort in humans because fluoride converts to hydrofluoric acid (HF) in the stomach. And "even at low concentrations HF can aggravate and prevent healing of ulcerated tissue".[63]

Imagine how fluoridated water can affect the inflamed, sensitive gut of IBD people.

Water Fluoridation is Banned in Europe

Did you know that in 97% of Western Europe, *adding fluoride to drinking water is illegal,* due to environmental and health concerns?

Citizens of the following countries drink non-fluoridated water: Austria, Belgium, Denmark, Finland, France, Germany, Greece, Iceland, Italy, Luxembourg, Netherlands, Northern Ireland, Norway, Portugal, Scotland, Sweden, Switzerland, and around 90% of the United Kingdom and Spain.[64]

Sadly, this toxic fluoride is still added to drinking water in the United States. Let's hope that in the future the U.S. will follow the EU Health Authority's decision on water fluoridation.

If you think you can avoid industrial fluoride by drinking bottled water, think again. I was shocked to learn that many brands of bottled water sold in the U.S. contain fluoride.

Check http://knowyourgut.com/resources for more info on fluoride-safe brands of water – and brands to avoid.

Chlorine in Your Water Wipes Out Beneficial Gut Flora

Water utilities add chlorine to over 98% of all drinking water in the U.S., because chlorine effectively kills harmful microorganisms that can cause dysentery, cholera, and typhoid fever. Sadly, chlorine destroys not only pathogens in your drinking water, but also beneficial bacteria in your gut.

Furthermore, studies show that chlorinated water increases your risk of bladder and colon cancer. When chlorine combines with organic substances in water, it produces chloramine. According to an American Journal of Public Health study, chlorinated water accounted for 6,500 new cases of rectal cancer and 4,200 cases of bladder cancer in the United States. Currently, colon cancer affects more than 140,000 Americans each year.[65]

Also, here is another scary fact. When added to water, chlorine combines with disinfection by-products and organic matter naturally occurring in the water - this combination produces trihalomethanes (THM). These toxic compounds are considered Group B carcinogens. They are trichloromethane (chloroform), dibromochloromethane, bromodichloromethane, and tribromomethane (bromoform).[66]

Recommendation: If you don't have a water filter, you can remove chlorine from your water for free. Just fill a large pot with water and leave it in the open air for at least 24 hours - most of the chlorine will evaporate. However, keep in mind that other contaminants will stay in the water.

Heavy Metals in Water are Linked to Immune System Damage

It's a fact that our exposure to heavy metals (e.g., lead, mercury, and arsenic) through water, food, and soil has a devastating effect on our health and immune system. Let's look at these heavy metals.

Lead

Research links lead exposure to numerous health problems, including damage to the immune system. If you have been exposed to lead contamination, you may experience abdominal pain, asthma, joint and muscle pain, kidney damage, and fertility problems. A high blood level of lead interferes with your body's ability to produce hemoglobin, which can result in anemia. The EPA states that lead exposure in children results in lowered IQ, nervous system damage, and learning disabilities.

Lead from street pipes may contaminate water in your plumbing. You should practice "flushing" - run your water for at least 3-5 minutes before use to decrease the lead content. Then, this "flushed" water must be filtered with a good home filter, to ensure that lead is removed completely.

Mercury

Mercury gets into soil and water from industrial water waste, fertilizers, fungicides, and coal-burning power plants. Small mercury particles are released into air via smoke, and they then enter our water and soil. About 30% of U.S. lakes and 25% of U.S. rivers contain enough mercury to cause a variety of health problems. Ingested mercury can cause bloody diarrhea, abdominal pain, ulcers, and IBD. Mercury is known to destroy intestinal flora, which is associated with the body's reduced resistance to various infections.[67]

Moreover, mercury can have a devastating effect on the immune system by suppressing immunity and causing autoimmune syndrome.[67]

Arsenic

Arsenic is used to manufacture lead-acid batteries, computer chips, insecticides, and wood preservatives. Contaminated drinking water is a main source of human exposure to arsenic. In adults, chronic exposure to arsenic is linked to depression and memory loss. Acute exposure to arsenic may cause diarrhea, nausea, vomiting, bloody urine, skin ulcers, kidney failure, and increased risk of getting sick with cancer of the prostate, bladder, kidney, lung, and skin.[68]

The Ugly Truth about Bottled Water

If you think that bottled water is better than tap, think again. According to the Environmental Working Group (EWG) "bottled water contains disinfection byproducts, fertilizer residue, and pain medication." They tested 10 popular brands of bottled water purchased from retail stores in California, Virginia, Delaware, North Carolina, Maryland, and District of Columbia. Laboratory tests confirmed that the tested bottled water "contained 38 chemical pollutants altogether, with an average of 8 contaminants in each brand."

So, what is going on with bottled water?

The EWG states:

> *"Unlike tap water, where consumers are provided with test results every year, the bottled water industry is not required to disclose the results of any contaminant testing that is conducted. Instead, the industry hides behind the claim that bottled water is held to the same safety standards as tap water. But with promotional campaigns saturated with images of mountain springs, and prices 1,900 times the price of tap water, consumers are clearly led to believe that they are buying a product that has been purified to a level beyond the water that comes out of the garden hose.*
>
> *To the contrary, our tests strongly indicate that the purity of bottled water cannot be trusted. Given the industry's refusal to make available data to support their claims of superiority, consumer confidence in the purity of bottled water is simply not justified."*[69]

Recommendation: If you must drink bottled water while traveling, look for imported water from Europe, because all bottled water in the EU is strictly regulated under EU law. Some examples of European imported water available in the U.S. are Voss, Hildon, Volvic, Evian, Icelandic, Panna, Gerolsteiner, and Perrier.

Clean Water Solution

If you eat a super clean diet, and still drink unfiltered, chlorinated, fluoridated tap water, or even some brands of bottled water, you are compromising your health. The human body is composed of about 60% water, which is used by all tissues, organs, and cells. Your body loses water when you digest food, when you sweat, and when you breathe. So, drinking clean water is essential to maintaining the healthy functions of your body.

So, start drinking clean, filtered water free of fluoride, heavy metals, and pathogens. To understand what type of contaminants are in your tap water, you can start with checking out the EWG's guide to Tap Water Database by entering your ZIP code.

Here is the link: https://www.eg.org/tapwater/

If you have your own well, you should test your water for heavy metal toxicity, bacteria, and chemicals. Ideally, after you complete your investigation on water purity and quality in your home, research home water filtration/purification systems. Keep in mind that your water filtration system should be able to filter out not only chemicals, harmful bacteria, and toxins, but also fluoride. Don't cut corners; inexpensive pour-through carbon pitchers are inadequate in removing municipal water contaminants such as fluoride and PFAS (perfluorooctanoic acid, used in chemical and industrial processing).

At first, I thought that installing a water filter was too expensive. Then, I calculated how much money I spend a year on bottled water. I realized that, in the long run, even an expensive filter will be much cheaper than regularly buying bottled water.

Plus, after you are done with drinking bottled water, all the glass and plastic containers remain and must be recycled. It takes hundreds of years for plastic water bottles to decompose. This plastic pollution ends up in our air, water, and food, in the form of tiny plastic particles.

I have installed a water filter in my house - however, I am reluctant to recommend any specific system due to ever-changing technology. Just do research and make sure that your filter can filter out pathogenic bacteria, parasites, heavy metals, chlorine, pesticides, herbicides, and fluoride.

Environmental Toxins

Is Your Environment Poisoning You and Contributing to Your Sickness?

Environmental toxins may contribute to IBD in two ways, according to WebMD:

1. "Toxins may trigger an immune system response."
2. "Toxins may directly damage the lining of the intestines. This may cause Crohn's disease to begin or to speed up." [70]

Plastic, Plastic Everywhere

If you look around your kitchen and fridge, you will see so many items that are made of plastic. Plastic water bottles, plastic food containers, plastic grocery bags, plastic wrap, plastic food bowls, plastic cups, plastic forks and knives, etc.

Crude oil and chemical compounds (plasticizers, stabilizers and artificial colorings) are used to manufacture plastic. Plastic products may leach chemicals into your food or water under the following conditions:

- When scratched
- When heated in a microwave
- When repeatedly washed in a dishwasher
- When coming in contact with fatty foods (e.g. butter, bacon, avocado) or acidic foods (e.g. tomato juice, yogurt, pickled veggies)[71]

BPA is Linked to Severe IBD Symptoms

Bisphenol A (BPA) is used in manufacturing of plastic food containers, water bottles, baby bottles, and lining of canned foods and drinks.

BPA can leach into food and beverages from containers made with this chemical.

According to the National Institute of Environmental Health Sciences (NIEHS), BPA is a known toxin and "endocrine disruptor" that is known to imitate estrogen, which triggers harmful changes in the endocrine system. Also, "these chemicals are linked with developmental, reproductive, brain, immune, and other problems."[72]

For years, research has linked BPA to cancer and infertility. Now, new research is linking BPA to worsening of ulcerative colitis symptoms in mice, increasing intestinal inflammation, and even mortality.

A study published in 2018 in the Journal of Experimental Biology and Medicine showed that female mice exposed daily to BPA for only 15 days suffered from acute intestinal inflammation and rectal bleeding. This study was by Dr. Kimberly Allred, a leading researcher from Texas A&M University.

Dr. Kimberly Allred states:

> *"The number of new cases of IBD are increasing, especially in nations that become more industrialized. While the causes of IBD have not yet been determined, several risk factors for developing it or worsening symptoms have been suggested. One such risk factor, the hormone estrogen, has been linked with an increased risk of IBD - and BPA can act as an estrogen. Furthermore, BPA has been previously shown to alter gut microbes similarly to the way the gut microbiota is altered in IBD patients."*[73]

How can you know which products contain BPA?

Just look at the bottom of a bottle or container - if you see a stamp of a triangle with the number 7, this container is very likely to contain BPA. Please note that canned foods can also contain BPA. So, instead of canned, try to use more fresh or frozen foods.

What can you use instead of plastic?

After I learned about the danger of plastic products, I got rid of most of the plastic in my kitchen. I purchased glass storage containers, glass measuring cups, and glass jars to store herbs, whole grain, and nuts. I also bought wooden cutting boards, stainless steel forks and knives, and ceramic plates and bowls.

Instead of plastic water bottles, I use glass bottles instead. I have 2 water bottles made from glass, so I always carry 1 or 2 with me. I don't like stainless steel bottles because after a while they retain food and drink residue and become discolored and hard to wash.

Learn the Plastic Code

Learn the numbers stamped on the bottom of your plastic bottles and containers, so you can make informed decisions for yourself and your loved ones. Below are some of the numbers and what they mean.

Relatively Safe Plastics

If you must use plastic, here are some are relatively safe plastics to hold water and food:

- #1 (PETE: polyethylene terephthalate) used in water and soft drink bottles
- #2 (HDPE: high-density polyethylene) used in milk containers and vitamin bottles
- #4 (LDPE: low-density polyethylene) used in product packaging and shopping bags
- #5 (PP: polypropylene) used in cream cheese, yogurt, containers, and kitchenware

In general, these plastics are considered safe; however repeated use/ washing will degrade the plastic and release toxins.

Steer clear of plastic containers with these labels:

- #3 (V: polyvinyl chloride)
- #6 (PS: polystyrene)
- #7 (OTHER or O)

Styrene is an industrial chemical that is used to produce Styrofoam products, plastic drinking cups, plates and containers. Some of the styrene can be transferred from the plastic container into some food or beverage.

Beware of Styrofoam products!

Styrene is an industrial chemical that is used to produce Styrofoam products, plastic drinking cups, plates and containers.

According to the Safe Drinking Water and Toxic Enforcement Act of California, "styrene is on the Proposition 65 list because it can cause cancer". Proposition 65 has a list of chemicals known to cause cancer and reproductive problems.[74]

How do you get exposed to styrene?

Some of the styrene can be transferred from the plastic container into some food or beverage. So, when you get hot coffee, tea, or cocoa in those cute white Styrofoam cups or when you pop a Styrofoam takeout container in the microwave to reheat your food, remember - you are drinking and eating cancer-causing chemicals.

How to reduce your exposure to plastics and BPA

- Stop cooking food in plastic bags or containers. It became popular to cook grains like rice and buckwheat or vegetables in prepackaged plastic bags, but don't do it! During cooking, the plastic residues may leach into your food, dramatically increasing your exposure to health-damaging chemicals.

- Don't reheat food in plastic in the microwave. Use the stovetop and a Teflon-free pan to heat your leftovers.
- Use glass Tupperware and glass mason jars to store leftover food, peeled veggies, fruits, and sprouts.
- Carry your own glass bottle filled with spring water or filtered water.
- Cut down on the amount of canned food you eat. Use more fresh or frozen foods, instead of canned.
- Whenever you must take hot drinks to go, ask for paper cups instead of plastic or Styrofoam.

Toxins in Personal Care and Home Products

Skin is our largest organ. It works as a protective barrier against invading germs, dehydration, cold, and heat. When we sweat, skin also excretes toxins from our body via our pores.

Have you ever used therapies that deliver drugs through the skin, such as skin patches for lower back pain? Or nicotine patches to help stop smoking? Consider that these drugs work faster than a pill taken by mouth. This is because whatever you put on your skin goes directly into your bloodstream. Therefore, protecting your skin against harsh chemicals is as important as eating a healthy diet.

NYS Health Foundation published a report that states:

> *"Everyday personal care products, such as cosmetics and shampoo, can contain chemicals associated with asthma, allergies, hormone disruption, neurodevelopmental problems, infertility, and even cancer. Americans use an average of 10 personal care products each day. The average person in the United States is exposed to chemicals from*

cosmetics, shampoo, and other personal care products before leaving the house each morning."

"According to the Environmental Working Group, the 12,500 unique chemical ingredients in these products equate to about one of every seven of the 82,000 chemicals registered for use in the U.S. Personal care products contain carcinogens, pesticides, reproductive toxins, endocrine disruptors, plasticizers, degreasers, and surfactants. Exposure to personal care products typically begins in infancy, with products such as baby shampoo and diaper cream, and continues throughout the lifespan."[75]

Just think, how many chemicals are absorbed through your skin when you:

- Use soap, shampoo, toothpaste, body wash, conditioner, antiperspirants, styling gel, or hair spray?
- Apply moisturizers, foundation, facial cream, eye cream, eye liner, mascara, nail polish, blush, or lipstick?
- Put on perfumes, colognes, shaving creams, sunscreen, tanning spray, or bug spray?

Check your personal care and home products for the following:

#1 Parabens

Like BPA, parabens are endocrine-disrupting chemicals. They are synthetic preservatives that are added to makeup, hair care products, deodorants, toothpaste, shampoo, conditioners, body lotions, and shaving products. These preservatives are used to extend products' shelf life and to prevent growth of harmful bacteria and fungus.

Exposure to Parabens is linked to Immune Dysfunction and Cancer

"The non-profit Campaign for Safe Cosmetics (CSC) reports that parabens mimic estrogen by binding to estrogen receptors on cells.

Research has shown that the perceived influx of estrogen beyond normal levels can in some cases trigger reactions such as increasing breast cell division and the growth of tumors. CSC cites a 2004 British study that detected traces of 5 parabens in breast tumours of 19 out of 20 women studied. CSC reports that parabens have also been linked to reproductive, immunological, neurological and skin irritation problems."[76]

The European Union banned parabens in 2012.

Parabens can be listed on the label as:

- Benzylparaben
- Propylparaben
- Methylparaben
- Ethylparaben
- Butylparaben
- Alkyl parahydroxy benzoates

#2 Formaldehyde

Formaldehyde is a gas that is used as a preservative. It's classified as "known to be a human carcinogen" by the National Toxicology program and by the International Agency for Research on Cancer (IArC). Formaldehyde has been linked to increased risk of leukemia and brain cancer.[77]

The following products may contain formaldehyde: soap, baby shampoo, body wash, nail polish, nail polish remover, salon hair-straightening products, laundry, and dish detergent.[78]

Formaldehyde can be listed on the label as:

- DMDM Hydantoin
- Diazolidinyl Urea
- Imidazolidinyl Urea
- Quaternium 15
- Bronopol (2-bromo-2-nitropropane-1,3-diol)

- Hydroxymethylglycinate
- Formalin
- Formic aldehyde
- Methanediol
- Methanal
- Methyl aldehyde
- Methylene glycol
- Methylene oxide

#3 Phthalates

Phthalates are chemicals made from petroleum, used to make plastic more flexible. Phthalates can interfere with our endocrine system. Exposure to phthalates has been linked to problems with the female & male reproductive systems (including DNA damage to sperm), obesity, increased risk of ADHD in children, and cancer.[78]

The following products may contain phthalates: shampoo, soap, aftershave, perfumes, hair sprays, cosmetics, nail polish, skin moisturizers, perfumes, air fresheners, infant care products, plastic toys and vinyl products (shower curtains, inflatable mattresses, floorings, wallpaper), air fresheners, & food and drink containers.

Phthalates can be listed on the label as:

- BBP (Butyl benzyl phthalate)
- DBP (Di-n-butyl phthalate) DEHP (Di(2-ethylhexyl) phthalate)
- DIDP (Di-isodecyl phthalate)
- DINP (Diisononyl phthalate)
- DnHP (Di-n-hexyl phthalate)

Phthalates in Medications and Nutritional Supplements

Phthalates are added to the enteric coating of some medications and nutritional supplements. The enteric coating is designed to make the product break down slowly in your digestive system. If a medication or product label says, “time released” or “enteric coated”, then this product may contain phthalates. Talk to your doctor and pharmacist to check whether your drug or supplement contains phthalates.

Did you know that Asacol®, an anti-inflammatory medication for treating ulcerative colitis is covered with an enteric coating of dibutyl phthalate (DBP)? This coating prevents the breakdown of medication before it reaches the small intestine.

A 2004 study examined a urine sample from a man after he took Asacol® for 3 months. The results were shocking. The concentration of phthalates in his urine significantly exceeded the 95th percentile for males, as reported by the CDC in the general population.[79]

How to reduce your exposure to the above chemicals?

- Check ewg.org for chemical-free, personal care products, cosmetics, sunscreens, and healthy household cleaning products.
- Buy personal care products labeled “paraben-free”. They will often contain natural preservatives such as essential oils, vitamins, and glycerin.
- Avoid formaldehyde by checking out EWG’s Skin Deep Cosmetics Database. “It contains information on more than 77,000 products and their ingredients.”[80]
- Choose products labeled “phthalate-free” or “fragrance-free”.
- Use glass containers instead of plastic.
- Avoid reheating food in plastic containers, especially in a microwave.
- Drink water from glass bottles, NOT from plastic bottles.
- Replace vinyl shower curtains with nylon. Nylon is resistant to mold and dries quickly.

The Bottom Line: I do not suggest living on an isolated island to avoid all toxins at all times. However, we can try to limit our exposure to toxins by making smart choices in daily living. I promise you, these changes will help you create a healthier body, and will positively impact your quality of life.

Toxins in Your Cookware

So now, you are eating mostly organic food, drinking filtered water, and using pure personal care and home products. You feel ahead of the toxin-free game in your modern life. Sadly, there is one hidden source of toxins that you might be using multiple times a day. And it's hiding in your cookware.

Many people don't realize that cookware can be a source of toxicity. Did you know that nonstick pots, pans, and aluminum cookware can leach harsh chemicals into your food, causing multiple health problems like immune system dysfunction, nervous system damage, and even cancer?

Healthy, non-toxic cookware is a must for healthy cooking

It took me many years of trial and error to figure out which pots, pans, and bakeware are safe, practical, and good for my health. I want to share with you my 40 years of experience on using different types of cookware.

Non-Stick: Teflon and PTFE

When I came to the U.S., I was fascinated with nonstick cookware, especially when cooking omelets. I could use very little oil, and my omelet would slide off so easily from my nonstick pan, right onto my plate. And cleaning was a snap. It was only years later that I learned that nonstick pots and pans are coated with Teflon®, which is a polymer developed by DuPont. This polymer contains a chemical called PFOA (perfluorooctanoic acid).

In 2005, EPA scientists recommended PFOA be labelled a "likely carcinogen", which is a substance that can cause cancer in humans. These recommendations were based on studies that linked PFOA to multiple cancers in lab animals.[81]

After I learned about the dangers of PFOA, I got rid of my entire Teflon-coated cookware set.

Aluminum is Toxic

The first tea kettle that I bought in my teens was made from aluminum. I just loved how light it was and how quickly the water boiled. Years later, I learned from an independent test that an aluminum tea kettle can leach up to 6.7 mg of aluminum per liter of water.[82]

Aluminum cookware and baking pans can also leach aluminum directly into your food when you cook acidic foods like tomato sauce or when you cook or bake for hours, increasing the duration of food contact with aluminum.

Aluminum is a heavy metal and is considered neurotoxic. When ingested through food and water, over time, it can accumulate in your bones, kidneys, liver, and brain. This becomes a contributing factor to many symptoms and diseases, according to Dr. Ray Psonak from Environmental Health Care in Maine.

He lists symptoms and illnesses of excessive aluminum exposure, such as "headache, cognitive problems, learning disabilities, fatigue, bone pain, decreased bone density, ringing in the ears, gastrointestinal disorders, colic, hyperactivity, poor balance, degenerative muscular conditions, cancer, Alzheimer's dementia, low hemoglobin, low phosphorus, and elevated ammonia levels."[83]

So, I ditched my aluminum tea kettle, and bought a glass one instead. Also, I stopped using aluminum foil for baking in my kitchen. Instead, I use unbleached parchment paper for baking and roasting meat, fish, and veggies.

You should know that aluminum cookware is not the main source of our exposure to this toxic heavy metal. Harmful aluminum is found in an alarming number of foods, medications, and personal care products.

Aluminum in Foods

You might be surprised to learn that aluminum is used as an emulsifying agent in cheese spread and processed cheese.

Also, store-bought pickles may have added alum, which is aluminum salt (potassium aluminum sulfate or aluminum sulfate). It's done to create crisp and crunchy pickles. Make your own pickles to avoid ingesting aluminum.

Be aware that drinks and foods are packaged in pouches which are often laminated with aluminum. Self-rising flour, dough, cake mix, chocolate mix pouches, and even the much-loved juice pouches may contain aluminum.

Coffee creamers such as Coffee Mate may contain sodium aluminosilicate. Baking powder may contain sodium aluminum sulfate.

Food can also harbor additives containing aluminum. "The following additives contain aluminum compounds: E173, E520, E521, E523 E541, E545, E554, E555 E556, E559, bauxite (Aluminum dioxide)"[83]

Aluminum in Medications

According to the CDC, "an average adult in the United States eats about 7-8 mg of aluminum per day in their food." However, if you are taking certain medications, the amount you ingest could be 20 times higher than what average American adult eats.[84]

For example: "Antacids have 300-600 mg aluminum hydroxide (approximately 104-208 mg of aluminum) per tablet, capsule, or 5 milliliter (mL) liquid dose." Some aluminum-containing antacids include Maalox, Mylanta, Amphojel, Gaviscon Tablets, Nephrox, Acid Gone, and Genaton.

"Buffered aspirin may contain 10-20 mg of aluminum per tablet."[84]

Also, anti-diarrheal and pain relief medications can contain aluminum.

Aluminum in Personal Care Products

Antiperspirants often contain aluminum chlorohydrate to block underarm sweat. You can find aluminum in toothpaste (aluminum oxyhydroxide), shampoos, lotions, and sunscreens.

Silicone

Silicone kitchenware is popular because it's flexible, non-stick, and easy to clean. But is silicone safe for high temperature cooking? Some say it is safe, inert material that will not leach chemicals into food. However, some studies demonstrate that low molecular weight silicone particles can migrate into food containing fat.[85]

According to a 2015 study done in the Institute of Organic Chemistry, in Heidelberg University in Germany, long-term exposure to silicone can become a potential health hazard that can contribute to increased levels of inflammation in the body.[86]

After reading the studies, I became concerned about silicone particles in my food. So, for now, I have decided to avoid using silicone for baking and stove top cooking.

Toxin-free Kitchen Tools: What I use in my Kitchen

Now, you have learned about possible toxins hiding in your cookware. The tips below will give you an idea on what you can use safely in your kitchen.

You can find specific links to approved cookware at http://knowyourgut.com/resources.

Pots and Pans

Luckily, today we have wonderful healthy alternatives that we call "green" nonstick pots and pans. However, you should remember that some "healthy" cookware becomes "unhealthy" when it's chipped, cracked, or scratched, because it can leach toxic chemicals into your food.

In my kitchen, I use ceramic and porcelain coated pans, stainless steel pots, enameled pots, cast iron, and glass cookware. This environment-friendly and human-friendly cookware does not contain PTFE (polytetrafluoroethylene).

Enamel Coated Cast Iron

Enamel coated cast iron is traditional, classic cookware that I use all the time for stews, bone broths, and sauces. These pots work equally well for slow cooking in the oven, and on the stovetop. They don't react with acidic foods and do not need to be seasoned like cast iron pans, because the cast iron is glazed twice with enamel.

Enamel coated cast iron is great for roasting, pan-frying, braising, and sautéing. The 2 drawbacks are that this type of cookware is a bit heavy and tends to be expensive. However, if you buy a good quality item, it will last you for decades. I have had mine for 25 years.

Cast Iron Pans (Uncoated)

I recommend using cast iron pans for people with anemia. When you cook in this type of pan, a small amount of iron is released in your food, which can help increase your iron level. Make sure you properly season your new cast iron pan prior to using it.

How to Season a Cast Iron Pan:

- Wash the pan with hot water and soap. Rinse and dry fully.
- Apply a thin layer of grape seed oil to the inside and outside of the pan.
- Place a large cooking sheet on the bottom rack of the oven to catch oil drippings from the pan.
- Set oven temperature to 375 degrees F.

- Place the pan upside down on the middle rack of the oven.
- Bake the pan for 1 hour, then turn the oven off and let the pan cool completely.
- Voila! You have seasoned your pan.

Glass

Glass is my favorite cookware because it is made of inert material. Glass does not react with any type of foods, including acidic foods. Another plus - your food can be cooked and stored in the fridge in the same glass container. That means less washing and cleaning in the kitchen. Also, glass cookware is durable - I have had my glass cookware since the late 80's.

One thing I do not recommend is buying new Pyrex glass cookware. When I used new Pyrex glass containers for baking, they shattered. I was shocked. It turns out, according to Consumer Reports, "in the early 90s, Corning, the company that invented Pyrex, started using soda lime silicate glass instead of borosilicate." Lab tests done by Consumer Reports concluded that "even at modest kitchen temperature, there is a definite possibility of thermal shock fracture" for soda lime glass cookware. Unfortunately, the new Pyrex glass cookware is not as durable and heat resistant as it once was according to a Consumer Reports video called "Glass bakeware that shatters."

Look for heat-resistant glassware made of borosilicate glass. This type of glass is highly durable, safe, and resistant to thermal shock.

Ceramic

In my kitchen, I have a few large ceramic-coated pots. They're lightweight, durable, non-stick, and super easy to clean. I prefer tempered glass lids, so you can see your food cooking without lifting the lid. Look for ceramic interiors free from PFOA, PTFE, lead, and cadmium.

Stainless Steel

I just love the shine of a new stainless-steel pot. I have used many stainless-steel pots in my kitchen, from very cheap to moderately expensive. However, be aware that manufacturers sometimes make stainless steel cookware rust-resistant by adding heavy metals like nickel and chromium to iron. And nickel can negatively affect health, causing allergic dermatitis in some people sensitive to this metal.[87]

How to buy nickel-free cookware

When you look at the bottom of a stainless-steel pot or pan, you may see a stamp with either 18/10 or 18/08. These numbers indicate how much chromium and nickel this alloy contains. The first number (18) indicates the percentage of chromium. The second number (10 or 8) indicates the nickel. If you are sensitive to nickel and want to buy nickel-free stainless-steel cookware, look for an 18/0 stamp on the bottom of the pot or pan.

When choosing stainless steel cookware, I recommend 5-ply stainless steel. What does that mean? The word "ply" simply means layers. So, "5-ply" means that the cookware is made of 5 layers of metal, which results in durable, stain-resistant, and easy to clean cookware that can last a lifetime.

My recommendation on stainless steel cookware:

- Stainless steel can be used for vegetable soups, quick stir fries, or boiling/steaming.
- Do not use acids like vinegar, lemon, or wine when cooking in stainless steel. Use glass or an enamel crock pot instead.
- Do not make long-simmer bone broth in stainless steel pots. It may corrode.
- If your stainless-steel cookware becomes damaged or heavily scratched, get rid of it.
- Do not cook acidic foods like tomato sauce in stainless steel pots. According to research published in the Journal of Agricultural and Food Chemistry, metals (nickel and chromium) can leach

into acidic food like tomato sauce when cooked in stainless steel pots.[87]

Tea Kettles

You may not realize that your tea kettle can release harmful chemicals into your boiling water. For example, metal tea kettles can leach nickel into your boiling water. Tea kettles with interiors glazed in ceramic may contain lead and cadmium. These heavy metals can leach into your boiling water.

So, what is the safest material for tea kettles? The answer is glass - specifically borosilicate glass, known for its quality and ability to withstand high heat without cracking.

When I need to heat up water quickly (in less than 5 minutes), I use a glass electric tea kettle with auto shut-off.

The Bottom Line: For your cooking needs and health considerations, use ceramic or porcelain coated pans, stainless steel pots, enameled pots, cast iron, enameled cast iron Dutch ovens, and borosilicate glass cookware for a safe, practical, and sustainable kitchen.

Electromagnetic Toxins/Pollution

In today's technologically advanced world, humans are constantly bombarded with invisible electromagnetic fields (EMFs) emitted by electrically charged objects.

Just consider all the gadgets you have in your home: Wi-Fi routers, cell phones, Bluetooth devices, computers, televisions, electric water heaters, microwaves, smart meters, security alarms, mobile phone chargers, mp3 docking stations, alarm clocks, baby monitors, and electric blankets.

How EMF affects Our Body

It is a scientifically proven fact that exposure to EMF adversely impacts your overall health, including your brain and other vital organs and systems. Moreover, EMF directly damages your immunity.

According to a study published in 2016 in Canadian Journal of Physiology and Pharmacology, electromagnetic field (EMF) emitted from a cell phone can directly damage the immune system in rats.

For 30 days, animals were exposed to EMF for just 1 hour. This exposure resulted in significant decrease in their immunoglobulin levels (IgA, IgE, IgM, and IgG)" of these animals. Immunoglobulins are antibodies that are generated by the immune system to fight infections, bacteria, fungi and parasites. Less immunoglobulins in the blood means that the immune system functions are suppressed and unable to effectively fight infection.[88]

This fact is hugely important for people afflicted with IBD, whose immune system is impaired to begin with. Therefore, any additional possible damage to our immune system from EMF should be avoided as much as possible. Because it can make the process of flare recovery more difficult.

To help you with a quick start on your flare recovery program, below is a short summary of some simple but important steps recommended for immediate limiting of exposure to harmful EMF during your recovery.

Of course, as mentioned earlier in this book, it is strongly recommended you take time off your work and other activities to allow your body to concentrate completely on healing itself. Therefore, the proposed limitations on usage of various EMF emitting devices (computer, phone, router, etc.) should not be overly difficult.

In order to speed up your flare recovery, I strongly urge you to implement these two simple, but fundamentally important, steps:

1. **Limit your exposure to computers and to your phone to a maximum of 3 hours a day, especially while doing this program.** This might seem difficult at the beginning. But trust me, in just 48 hours or so, you will notice a difference in your overall level of mental calm and stability. You are dieting now, so do yourself a favor - include in your diet some limitations on consumption of harmful EMF as well. You will not regret it.
2. **Before going to sleep (or if possible, during the daytime as well), turn off your WIFI router and cell phone.** You must remember that all your communication devices, unless turned off (in some cases even disconnected from power), are constantly beaming harmful EMF into your body. If done daily and consistently, you'll quickly notice a difference in your mental and emotional stability.

The Bottom Line: I know, just following these two simple steps might feel overwhelming at first. After all, our smart phones and computers are an integral part of our life. For some of us, these gadgets may even feel like a part of us. I bet you know at least one person who sleeps with a smartphone. That is a pretty intimate relationship, wouldn't you say?

Well, it would be funny - if it was not so devastating to our health. Just make time to read books on the subject, and you will surely agree with me.

These gadgets enable us to be more productive at work, as well as providing us with an incredible means to communicate and stay more socially connected. The advantages associated with the use of these devices are obvious.

So, is it possible to balance these advantages and disadvantages without compromising our health, or our business and life conveniences?

Fortunately, yes. Just a few simple changes in daily smartphone usage can significantly reduce exposure to harmful EMF.

Here are some small changes I have implemented in my life:

Based on a review of studies published up until 2011, the **International Agency for Research on Cancer (IARC)** has classified RF (radiofrequency)radiation as "possibly carcinogenic to humans," based on limited evidence of a possible increase in risk for brain tumors among cell phone users.[89]

Change #1: I stopped keeping my phone next to my head while talking after I learned that radiation beaming from wireless headphones and cell phones may increase my risk of brain damage and cancer. Instead, I use a speaker or wired headphones. I also turn off Bluetooth on my cell phone and in my car stereo settings.

Change #2: When I am not on the phone, I try not to keep my phone next to the place I work or rest. I keep my cell phone at least a yard away from me. If I need to check my phone, I get up and walk a little.

Change #3: I switch my phone off before going to bed (may be scary for some at the beginning). Just try it for yourself and see that there is life with your smartphone turned off.

For the sake of your sustainable health, please educate yourself on this vitally important subject.

You'll find educational links on EMFs at http://knowyourgut.com/resources.

The Bottom Line: It might be stressful and overwhelming to implement all these recommended changes all at once, so take your time. Every little bit helps.

It took me many years to gather and implement the changes I am talking about in this chapter. The famous expression "Rome wasn't built in a day" is applicable to the changes you are planning to undertake in your life.

To make so many changes in your life takes time, money, attention, and knowledge. You have a lifetime to build better habits and a cleaner environment for yourself and your loved ones.

Toxic Emotions/Stress

In addition to being physically exhausted during flares, people with IBD experience great psychological stress because they often feel overwhelmed and unequipped to handle their disease. Missed days at school, and the inability to work or take care of family creates emotions of fear, bitterness, regret, and helplessness.

I know what it feels like being trapped by your own body, stuck in the bathroom...unable to get kids ready for school, or get to your job on time for the morning meeting. The toxic emotions of guilt, resentment, and anger can give you an ulcer - literally.

Furthermore, toxic emotions and stress provoke adrenal dysfunction. This ongoing, chronic, emotional stress is literally making you sick by raising cortisol levels (aka "the stress hormone").

Continuous, elevated levels of cortisol have a devastating effect on your body and your gut, exhausting the immune system and allowing inflammation to get out of control.

An impaired immune system and uncontrollable inflammation are two main triggers for exacerbation of a flare in ulcerative colitis and Crohn's disease.

Your thoughts create emotions, and your emotions create chemicals

When you change your thoughts and your emotions, you change your gut biology. What you think, how you react to stress, and your ability to express your feelings all directly impact your gut health. Uncontrollable anxiety, depression, fear, and excessive worrying push your body to create chemicals that can wipe out the beneficial bacteria in your gut, triggering overgrowth of harmful bacteria.

Did you know that you can literally get an ulcer while exposed to prolonged stress and feelings of anger and despair? When we are under continuous stress, our stomach acid is greatly reduced, leading to poor digestion of proteins and an overgrowth of harmful bacteria that creates dysbiosis, leading to another IBD flare.

Your digestion is controlled by your emotions. Gastroenterologist, Anil Minocha, MD, author of *Natural Stomach Care*, states:

> *"The gut literally has a mind of its own, and it is intimately, almost instantaneously, connected with the one in our brain."*

So, to heal your gut fast, you should consider your state of mind. When you control your state of mind, you are in charge of your emotions. When you learn to master your emotions, you can reduce and even eliminate chronic inflammation in your body.

Stress can trigger or worsen IBD flares-ups

Dr. Bernstein from IBD Clinical and Research Centre, in Winnipeg, Canada conducted a study on 552 patients with ulcerative colitis or Crohn's disease. The findings confirmed that stress (or even perception of stress) worsens IBD symptoms. IBD patients had to complete surveys every 3 months for 1 year, stating flare-up symptoms, perceived stress, and stressful events in their life. The result of the study confirmed that high levels of stress in the prior 3-month period increased the risk of IBD flare more than twofold. 52% of patients who experienced flares reported a high stress level in the previous 3 months, compared to 29% of symptom-free patients. Dr. Bernstein concluded that perceived stress is associated with increased risk of IBD symptoms.[90]

Dr. Bernstein notes:

> *"the sympathetic nervous system, which jumps into action during times of stress, acts on the lining of the colon, and might exacerbate existing inflammation. There is also evidence that stress hormones may help harmful bacteria take up residence in the intestines, which might, in turn, affect symptoms during stress. If stress does trigger IBD symptoms in some people, then it's possible that learning better ways of managing stress would help stave off flare-ups."*[91]

The Bottom Line: when it comes to preventing IBD flares, how you react to stress is one of the important factors that you can control. Of course, I am not talking about absolute control over our emotions. It's normal and very human for us to get upset and to cry sometimes. However, focusing all your attention on the stress of your illness and the hardship of your life brings a lot of negative emotions. These emotions trigger physiological effects that predispose you to disease. You can actually make yourself sick with negative thoughts and self-limiting beliefs by releasing stress hormones like cortisol, epinephrine, and adrenaline. Chronic stress and feelings of fear, anxiety, helplessness, and depression can shut down your body's natural self-repair mechanisms and worsen symptoms of IBD. This creates a vicious cycle of more disease symptoms and more negative feelings.

On the other hand, positive thoughts have a relaxing effect on your nervous system and help your digestive system heal and repair by releasing hormones of happiness: endorphins, dopamine, and serotonin.

Empowering beliefs will help you to become confident, optimistic, and satisfied. Being happier may reduce pain, strengthen your immunity, and help you to live longer.

That is why, at the most stressful times in my life, I tried to see my glass half full instead of half empty. And when life gave me lemons, I managed to make lemonade by learning what my disease is and how to reverse it.

I am convinced that by staying calm during stressful situations, and by controlling your mind and your thought process, you can significantly reduce your risk for future IBD flares. This creates a feeling of being in control of your life and your destiny. After all, you are in charge of what you think and feel!

Also, part of my healing was learning to forgive people who mistreated me. Clinging to resentment and anger is like leaving a knife inside your bleeding gut. Destructive emotions and stinky thinking literally poison your body and make you sick. By forgiving people who did you wrong, you give yourself the chance to truly heal - both emotionally and physically. Emotional detoxification is as important as physical detoxification. Replace hidden anger, resentment, fear, and anxiety... with joy, forgiveness, hope, and appreciation. This will help us feel better and will aid in healing our gut and body.

Keep in mind: your positive emotional stability during flare-up recovery is crucial. It will allow your body to produce good hormones, and other chemicals necessary for healing and rebuilding new healthy gut cells.

In the next chapter, you will learn about another cause of IBD - pathogens.

References

[1] Dubeau MF, Iacucci M, Beck PL, Moran GW, Kaplan GG, Ghosh S, Panaccione R. "Drug-induced inflammatory bowel disease and IBD-like conditions." *Inflamm Bowel Dis.* 2013 Feb;19(2):445-56. doi: 10.1002/ibd.22990. PMID:22573536. https://www.ncbi.nlm.nih.gov/pubmed/22573536

[2] https://www.cdc.gov/drugresistance/pdf/threats-report/2019-ar-threats-report-508.pdf

[3] https://www.physiciansweekly.com/antibiotic-use-linked-to-ibd-in-prospective-cohort-study

[4] Long H Nguyen, MD et al. Antibiotic use and the development of inflammatory bowel disease: a national case-control study in Sweden. *The Lancet Gastroenterology & Hepatology.* August 17, 2020

[5] Martin MJ, Thottathil SE, Newman TB. "Antibiotics Overuse in Animal Agriculture: A Call to Action for Health Care Providers." *Am J Public Health.* 2015;105(12):2409-2410. doi:10.2105/AJPH.2015.302870 https://www.ncbi.nlm.nih.gov/pmc/articles/PMC4638249/

[6] https://ec.europa.eu/commission/presscorner/detail/en/IP_05_1687

[7] https://www.webmd.com/food-recipes/news/20100628/fda-antibiotics-in-livestock-affects-human-health

[8] https://www.cdc.gov/drugresistance/pdf/ar-threats-2013-508.pdf

[9] Becattini S, Taur Y, Pamer EG. "Antibiotic-Induced Changes in the Intestinal Microbiota and Disease." *Trends Mol Med.* 2016;22(6):458-478. doi:10.1016/j.molmed.2016.04.003

[10] https://www.physiciansweekly.com/antibiotic-use-linked-to-ibd-in-prospective-cohort-study/

[11] Nguyen, Long H et al. "Antibiotic use and the development of inflammatory bowel disease: a national case-control study in Sweden." *The Lancet. Gastroenterology & hepatology* vol. 5,11 (2020): 986-995. doi:10.1016/S2468-1253(20)30267-3

[12] Shaw SY, Blanchard JF, Bernsten CN "Association between the use of antibiotics and new diagnoses of Crohn's disease and ulcerative colitis." *Am J Gastroenterol.* 2011 Dec;106(12):2133-42. doi: 10.1038/ajg.2011.304. Epub 2011 Sep 13

[13] Khalili, Hamed. "Risk of Inflammatory Bowel Disease with Oral Contraceptives and Menopausal Hormone Therapy: Current Evidence and Future Directions." *Drug safety* vol. 39,3 (2016): 193-7. doi:10.1007/s40264-015-0372-y

[14] Long, Millie D.Hutfless, Susan et al. "Shifting Away From Estrogen-Containing Oral Contraceptives in Crohn's Disease." *Gastroenterology*, April 29, 2016 Volume 150, Issue 7, 1518 – 152

[15] Khalili H, Higuchi LM, Ananthakrishnan AN, Richter JM, Feskanich D, Fuchs CS, Chan AT. "Oral contraceptives, reproductive factors and risk of inflammatory bowel disease." *Gut.* 2013 Aug;62(8):1153-9. doi: 10.1136/gutjnl-2012-302362. Epub 2012 May 22. https://www.ncbi.nlm.nih.gov/pmc/articles/PMC3465475/

[16] https://health.usnews.com/health-news/news/articles/2012/05/21/birth-control-pills-hrt-tied-to-digestive-ills

[17] American College of Gastroenterology (ACG) 2011 Annual Scientific Meeting and Postgraduate Course. Abstract #6. Presented October 31, 2011. https://www.medscape.com/viewarticle/752846

[18] Felder, J B et al. "Effects of nonsteroidal antiinflammatory drugs on inflammatory bowel disease: a case-control study." *The American journal of gastroenterology* vol. 95,8 (2000): 1949-54. doi:10.1111/j.1572-0241.2000.02262.x https://pubmed.ncbi.nlm.nih.gov/10950041

[19] https://www.drugwatch.com/accutane/lawsuits/

[20] https://www.northjersey.com/story/news/new-jersey/2017/01/24/nj-supreme-court-reinstates-25m-verdict-accutane-case/97001490/

[21] https://law.justia.com/cases/new-jersey/appellate-division-unpublished/1988/a3280-07-opn.html

[22] http://digestivemedicalsolutions.com/the-good-the-bad-and-the-ugly-side-of-gmos-and-their-link-to-ibd

[23] https://www.aaemonline.org/aaem-calls-for-immediate-moratorium-on-genetically-modified-foods/

[24] https://chiro.org/nutrition/FULL/Genetically_Modified_Foods_Warning.shtml

[25] https://responsibletechnology.org/docs/state_science_gmo.pdf

[26] https://www.gmoseralini.org/faq-items/why-this-study-now/
Séralini, Gilles-Eric et al. "Republished study: long-term toxicity of a Roundup herbicide and a Roundup-tolerant genetically modified maize." *Environmental sciences* Europe vol. 26,1 (2014): 14. doi:10.1186/s12302-014-0014-5

[27] Judy A. Carman, Howard R. Vlieger, Larry J. Ver Steeg, Verlyn E. Sneller, Garth W. Robinson, Catherine A. Clinch-Jones, Julie I. Haynes, John W. Edwards (2013). "A long-term toxicology study on pigs fed a combined genetically modified (GM) soy and GM maize diet." *Journal of Organic Systems* 8 (1): 38-54.

[28] Ananthakrishnan, Ashwin N et al. "Long-term intake of dietary fat and risk of ulcerative colitis and Crohn's disease." *Gut* vol. 63,5 (2014): 776-84. doi:10.1136/gutjnl-2013-305304 https://www.ncbi.nlm.nirah.gov/pmc/articles/PMC3915038/

[29] Kaliannan, Kanakaraju et al. "A host-microbiome interaction mediates the opposing effects of omega-6 and omega-3 fatty acids on metabolic endotoxemia." *Scientific reports* vol. 5 11276. 11 Jun. 2015, doi:10.1038/srep11276 https://www.ncbi.nlm.nih.gov/pubmed/26062993

[30] A.P. Simopoulos. "Evolutionary aspects of diet, the omega-6/omega-3 ratio and genetic variation: nutritional implications for chronic diseases". *Biomedicine & Pharmacotherapy* Volume 60, Issue 9, November 2006, Pages 502-507. https://www.sciencedirect.com/science/article/abs/pii/S0753332206002435

[31] https://www.worldatlas.com/articles/top-sugar-consuming-nations-in-the-world.html

[32] https://www.dhhs.nh.gov/dphs/nhp/documents/sugar.pdf

[33] Buyken, Anette E et al. "Carbohydrate nutrition and inflammatory disease mortality in older adults." The *American journal of clinical nutrition* vol. 92,3 (2010): 634-43. doi:10.3945/ajcn.2010.29390
https://pubmed.ncbi.nlm.nih.gov/20573797/

[34] Xiaofa Qin, MD, PhD. "How Sugar and Soft Drinks Are Related to Inflammatory Bowel Disease?" *Inflammatory Bowel Diseases*, Volume 22, Issue 6, 1 June 2016, Pages E18–E19, https://doi.org/10.1097/MIB.0000000000000774
https://academic.oup.com/ibdjournal/article/22/6/E18/4561887

[35] University of Alberta Faculty of Medicine & Dentistry. "Sugar binges increase risk of inflammatory bowel disease." ScienceDaily. *ScienceDaily*, 14 November 2019. http://www.sciencedaily.com/releases/2019/11/191114115949.htm

[36] https://livingnongmo.org/2018/06/25/gmo-feature-sugar-beets/

[37] Case Western Reserve University. "Artificial sweetener could intensify symptoms in those with Crohn's disease: Promotes 'bad' bacteria and intestinal inflammation; findings may guide dietary habits in human patients." *ScienceDaily*, 15 March 2018. http://www.sciencedaily.com/releases/2018/03/180315155411.htm

[38] Abou-Donia, Mohamed B et al. "Splenda alters gut microflora and increases intestinal p-glycoprotein and cytochrome p-450 in male rats." *Journal of toxicology and environmental health*. Part A vol. 71,21 (2008): 1415-29. doi:10.1080/15287390802328630
https://www.ncbi.nlm.nih.gov/pubmed/18800291

[39] Qin, Xiaofa. "Etiology of inflammatory bowel disease: a unified hypothesis." *World journal of gastroenterology* vol. 18,15 (2012): 1708-22. doi:10.3748/wjg.v18.i15.1708
https://www.ncbi.nlm.nih.gov/pmc/articles/PMC3332284/

[40] Mäkinen, Kauko K. "Gastrointestinal Disturbances Associated with the Consumption of Sugar Alcohols with Special Consideration of Xylitol: Scientific Review and Instructions for Dentists and Other Health-Care Professionals." *International journal of dentistry* vol. 2016 (2016): 5967907. doi:10.1155/2016/5967907
https://www.ncbi.nlm.nih.gov/pmc/articles/PMC5093271/

[41] Deniņa, I et al. "The influence of stevia glycosides on the growth of Lactobacillus reuteri strains." *Letters in applied microbiology* vol. 58,3 (2014): 278-84. doi:10.1111/lam.12187
https://www.ncbi.nlm.nih.gov/pubmed/24251876

[42] CSPI Says Food Dyes Pose Rainbow of Risks: Cancer, Hyperactivity, Allergic Reactions. June 29, 2010 https://cspinet.org/new/201006291.html

[43] Vojdani, Aristo, and Charlene Vojdani. "Immune reactivity to food coloring." *Alternative therapies in health and medicine* vol. 21 Suppl 1 (2015): 52-62. https://www.ncbi.nlm.nih.gov/pubmed/25599186

[44] https://www.ewg.org/foodscores/content/natural-vs-artificial-flavors

[45] Vally, Hassan, and Neil LA Misso. "Adverse reactions to the sulphite additives." *Gastroenterology and hepatology from bed to bench* vol. 5,1 (2012): 16-23.
https://www.ncbi.nlm.nih.gov/pmc/articles/PMC4017440/

[46] https://oehha.ca.gov/proposition-65/proposition-65-list

[47] https://www.cdc.gov/biomonitoring/Parabens_FactSheet.html

[48] Calafat, Antonia M et al. "Urinary concentrations of four parabens in the U.S. population: NHANES 2005-2006." *Environmental health perspectives* vol. 118,5 (2010): 679-85. doi:10.1289/ehp.0901560
https://www.ncbi.nlm.nih.gov/pmc/articles/PMC2866685/

[49] Salviano Dos Santos, Vânia Paula et al. "Benzene as a Chemical Hazard in Processed Foods." *International journal of food science* vol. 2015 (2015): 545640. doi:10.1155/2015/545640
https://www.ncbi.nlm.nih.gov/pmc/articles/PMC4745501/

[50] http://news.bbc.co.uk/2/hi/health/4465871.stm

[51] https://www.webmd.com/vitamins/ai/ingredientmono-1032/edta

[52] https://www.uofmhealth.org/health-library/d03951a1

[53] https://ntp.niehs.nih.gov/ntp/roc/content/listed_substances_508.pdf

[54] https://www.ewg.org/research/nearly-500-ways-make-yoga-mat-sandwich

[55] Fath, R B Jr et al. "Degraded carrageenan-induced colitis in CF1 mice. A clinical, histopathological and kinetic analysis." *Digestion* vol. 29,4 (1984): 197-203. doi:10.1159/000199033
https://pubmed.ncbi.nlm.nih.gov/6468767/

[56] Watt, J, and R Marcus. "Carrageenan-induced ulceration of the large intestine in the guinea pig." *Gut* vol. 12,2 (1971): 164-71. doi:10.1136/gut.12.2.164
https://pubmed.ncbi.nlm.nih.gov/5548564/

[57] http://natural-health-journals.com/gums-in-foods-causing-health-problems-for-many/

[58] https://wayback.archive-it.org/7993/20170112130913/
http:/www.fda.gov/NewsEvents/Newsroom/PressAnnouncements/ucm256253.htm

[59] Chassaing, Benoit et al. "Dietary emulsifiers impact the mouse gut microbiota promoting colitis and metabolic syndrome." *Nature* vol. 519,7541 (2015): 92-6. doi:10.1038/nature14232

https://www.ncbi.nlm.nih.gov/pmc/articles/PMC4910713/

[60] https://foodandnutrition.org/november-december-2017/food-additives-emulsifiers/

[61] Evans, Sydney et al. "Cumulative risk analysis of carcinogenic contaminants in United States drinking water." *Heliyon* vol. 5,9 e02314. 19 Sep. 2019, doi:10.1016/j.heliyon.2019.e02314

[62] https://www.scientificamerican.com/article/tap-drinking-water-contaminants-pollutants/

[63] Richard Sauerheber. "Physiologic Conditions Affect Toxicity of Ingested Industrial Fluoride". *Journal of Environmental and Public Health*. Volume 2013, Article ID 439490, 13 pages http://dx.doi.org/10.1155/2013/439490

[64] https://fluoridealert.org/content/europe-statements/

[65] https://www.nytimes.com/1992/07/01/us/tiny-cancer-risk-in-chlorinated-water.html

[66] https://water-research.net/index.php/trihalomethanes-disinfection

[67] Rice, Kevin M et al. "Environmental mercury and its toxic effects." *Journal of preventive medicine and public health = Yebang Uihakhoe* chi vol. 47,2 (2014): 74-83. doi:10.3961/jpmph.2014.47.2.74
https://www.ncbi.nlm.nih.gov/pmc/articles/PMC3988285/

[68] Judy E. Perkin. Metallic Environmental Contaminants: Behaviour & Nutrition

[69] Olga Naidenko, PhD et al. Bottled Water Quality Investigation. EWG, Oct 18, 2008

[70] https://www.webmd.com/ibd-crohns-disease/crohns-disease/qa/how-do-environmental-factors-cause-crohns-disease

[71] https://www.consumerreports.org/toxic-chemicals-substances/most-plastic-products-contain-potentially-toxic-chemicals/

[72] https://www.niehs.nih.gov/health/topics/agents/endocrine/index.cfm

[73] Texas A&M AgriLife Communications. "BPA risk factor for inflammatory bowel disease." *ScienceDaily*. ScienceDaily, 5 July 2018. www.sciencedaily.com/releases/2018/07/180705125720.htm

[74] https://www.p65warnings.ca.gov/fact-sheets/styrene

[75] Potentially Toxic Chemicals in Personal Care Products. NYS Health Foundation. https://nyshealthfoundation.org/wp-content/uploads/2019/03/potentially-toxic-chemicals-personal-care-products-march-2019.pdf

[76] https://www.scientificamerican.com/article/should-people-be-concerned-about-parabens-in-beauty-products/

[77] https://www.cancer.gov/about-cancer/causes-prevention/risk/substances/formaldehyde/formaldehyde-fact-sheet

[78] Potentially Toxic Chemicals in Personal Care Products. NYS Health Foundation. https://nyshealthfoundation.org/wp-content/uploads/2019/03/potentially-toxic-chemicals-personal-care-products-march-2019.pdf

[79] Betts, Kellyn S.. "Phthalates in Prescription Drugs: Some Medications Deliver High Doses." *Environmental Health Perspectives* vol. 117,2 (2009): A74.

[80] https://www.ewg.org/research/exposing-cosmetics-cover

[81] https://yosemite.epa.gov/sab/sabproduct.nsf/ded77e69fc8ced288525711e006fe16b/$file/kropp-ewg.pdf

[82] https://cookware.mercola.com/ceramic-teaware.aspx

[83] http://www.chelationmedicalcenter.com/aluminum-toxic-heavy-metal.html

[84] https://www.atsdr.cdc.gov/ToxProfiles/tp22-c1-b.pdf

[85] Helling, Ruediger et al. "Migration behaviour of silicone moulds in contact with different foodstuffs." *Food additives & contaminants. Part A, Chemistry, analysis, control, exposure & risk assessment* vol. 27,3 (2010): 396-405. doi:10.1080/19440040903341869

[86] Jürgen H. Gross. "Analysis of Silicones Released from Household Items and Baby Articles by Direct Analysis in Real Time-Mass Spectrometry". *J. Am. Soc. Mass Spectrom.* (2015) 26:511Y521 DOI: 10.1007/s13361-014-1042-5

[87] Kamerud, Kristin L et al. "Stainless steel leaches nickel and chromium into foods during cooking." *Journal of agricultural and food chemistry* vol. 61,39 (2013): 9495-501. doi:10.1021/jf402400v
https://www.ncbi.nlm.nih.gov/pmc/articles/PMC4284091/

[88] El-Gohary, Ola Ahmed, and Mona Abdel-Azeem Said. "Effect of electromagnetic waves from mobile phone on immune status of male rats: possible protective role of vitamin D." *Canadian journal of physiology and pharmacology* vol. 95,2 (2017): 151-156. doi:10.1139/cjpp-2016-0218
https://pubmed.ncbi.nlm.nih.gov/27901344/

[89] https://www.cancer.org/cancer/cancer-causes/radiation-exposure/cellular-phones.html

[90] Bernstein, Charles N et al. "A prospective population-based study of triggers of symptomatic flares in IBD." *The American journal of gastroenterology* vol. 105,9 (2010): 1994-2002. doi:10.1038/ajg.2010.140

[91] https://www.reuters.com/article/us-stress-trigger/stress-may-be-a-trigger-of-bowel-disease-symptoms-idUSTRE63F3AW20100416

CHAPTER 4

Infection-causing Pathogens are IBD triggers

Studies confirm that both colitis and Crohn's can be triggered by specific infectious agents/microorganisms like pathogenic bacteria, viruses, fungi, and parasites. These harmful bugs can burrow and literally eat away the delicate lining of your gastrointestinal tract, causing chronic inflammation and an abnormal immune response. Symptoms of intestinal infections are identical to IBD symptoms such as abdominal pain, fever, bloody diarrhea, and weight loss. These infections can start the IBD disease process and/or trigger an IBD flare.

The following infections are associated with IBD:

- Clostridium difficile bacteria causes C. difficile colitis
- MAP (Mycobacterium avium paratuberculosis) is associated with Crohn's disease
- E. coli (Escherichia coli) bacterial infection can mimic Crohn's disease symptoms of abdominal pain, nausea, diarrhea, and fever
- Salmonella or Campylobacter bacteria may contribute to ulcerative colitis
- Cytomegalovirus infection may contribute to ulcerative colitis flare
- Fungi is a key factor in the development of IBD (Crohn's and colitis)
- Parasite infection can mimic IBD (Crohn's and colitis)

Let's take a closer look at pathogens in IBD.

Bacteria and IBD Connection

Clostridium difficile bacteria causes C. difficile colitis

Clostridium difficile (also called C. diff) is aggressive, pathogenic bacteria that can irritate the large intestine and cause diarrhea, fever, and abdominal cramps. An infected person can spread C. diff if they don't wash their hands after using the bathroom, going on to prepare food, or touch different objects like a door handle, or a bed rail in a hospital or nursing home. This may leave C. diff bacteria spores in food, or on objects the infected person touched. That is how you can get infected: when you eat C. diff-contaminated food or touch a C. diff-contaminated object.

Also, you can get sick with C.diff when you take antibiotics to treat infection. Our intestines contain close to 2000 different bacteria, most of which protect your body from infection. However, when you take antibiotics, it wipes out both good and bad bacteria in your gut. Without good intestinal bacteria to protect you, C. diff can quickly grow out of control in your colon and release toxins, causing serious colon inflammation that results in C. diff colitis.[1]

C. diff infection can be misdiagnosed as ulcerative colitis because symptoms for both diseases are so similar (diarrhea, severe abdominal cramps, fever, weight loss).

MAP bacteria is associated with Crohn's and Ulcerative Colitis

MAP (Mycobacterium avium paratuberculosis) bacteria can cause tuberculosis (Mycobacterium tuberculosis). According to a study published in Gut Pathogens journal, MAP has been identified in humans as the main cause of Crohn's disease, and to lesser extent ulcerative colitis. MAP has been recovered

> *"From the blood of patients with Crohn's disease (55%) and ulcerative colitis (22%) but not from control subjects. Non-controlled studies have reported that up to 84% of patients respond to treatment with combinations of antibiotics effective against MAP."*[2]

You can get infected with MAP bacteria by eating infected beef and/or consuming dairy products from infected cows. You can also get infected by drinking poorly treated farm runoff water. Unfortunately, water filtration and chlorination do not fully eliminate MAP. Moreover, MAP can survive freezing, and can be found in an ice cream up to 1 year after the manufacturing date.[3]

The Bottom Line: It turns out standard milk pasteurization does not kill MAP bacteria. So, store-bought milk and yogurt can contain MAP bacteria.

If you have CD or UC, avoid all dairy products, especially during a flare.

Why is MAP bacteria not killed during pasteurization? During pasteurization, commercial milk is heated at 161°F (72°C) for only 15 seconds. For bacteria to be killed, milk must be boiled to 212°F (100°C).[4]

If you eat meat, it must be from grass-fed, healthy cows, and cooked long enough, or at a high enough temperature to kill bacteria.

E. coli infection can mimic Crohn's disease

E. coli (aka Escherichia coli) is a harmless bacteria that resides in the lower intestines of animals and humans. But there is an infectious strain called E. coli O157:H7 that produces Shiga toxin. This pathogenic E. coli strain enters your body when you eat infected food such as undercooked meat, fresh produce, raw milk, raw cheese, and other raw dairy products. Water can also become contaminated with E. coli.

This infectious E. coli strain is known to cause "traveler's diarrhea". Infected individuals will experience abdominal cramps, nausea, vomiting, fever, and severe diarrhea. Symptoms of infection with E. coli are similar to symptoms of Crohn's disease: abdominal pain and cramping, bloody diarrhea, fever and vomiting. About 265,000 people get sick with E. coli every year in the United States.[5]

According to Dr. Karel Geboes and Dr. Gert De Hertogh from University Hospital KU Leuven in Belgium,

> *"Escherichia coli bacteria infection can mimic CD clinically, radiologically and endoscopically. Differential diagnosis is done by stool culture."*[6]

In a 2004 study published in Gastroenterology Journal, 63 patients with Crohn's disease were examined for the presence of E. coli. The study revealed that:

> *"An invasive strain of E. coli was recovered from 22% of mucosal biopsies from Crohn's disease patients with chronic, postoperative, recurrent inflammation in the ileum."*[7]

Stool samples are used to diagnose E. coli infection and its toxins. It's not recommended to take anti-diarrheal medications if you have this bacterial infection, as it may hinder your body's ability to eliminate E. coli and its toxins and may delay your recovery. Moreover, according to microbiologist Sarah Fankhauser, at Emory University in Georgia, E. coli infections in the intestinal tract should not be treated with antibiotics because:

> *"Antibiotics may kill other beneficial bacteria in the gut, allowing more space and nutrients for the E. coli to grow."*

Antibiotics *are* recommended if a person has a UTI (urinary tract infection) caused by E. coli.[8]

Important Comment:

Do not swallow water when swimming in freshwater (e.g., lakes and rivers). These bodies of water can harbor E. coli. One of my clients got sick with infectious colitis caused by E. coli, after falling into a lake and swallowing the contaminated freshwater.

Private wells can also be a source of E. coli bacteria. If you have a private well, make sure to boil your water for at least 5 minutes. When you travel, especially outside of the U.S., do not drink tap water, use ice, or eat raw fruits and vegetables that have been washed with tap water. You can prevent E. coli infection by washing and disinfecting all fresh fruits and vegetables, and cooking meats to proper internal temperatures.

Salmonella or Campylobacter Infections increase Risk for IBD

You can get sick with Salmonella or Campylobacter bacteria after drinking raw, contaminated milk or by eating undercooked meat, poultry, or shellfish. Infected people develop abdominal cramps, fever, and diarrhea.

Salmonella and Campylobacter infections are common.

"CDC estimates that Salmonella causes about 1.2 million illnesses and Campylobacter causes an estimated 1.3 million illnesses each year in the US; most likely due to eating raw or undercooked poultry, or to eating something that touched it." [9, 10]

Danish researchers Gradel and Nielsen conducted a study comparing 13,148 patients with Salmonella/Campylobacter gastroenteritis vs. 26,216 individuals without infection. The study duration was for 15 years from 1991 through 2003. It turns out that getting sick with Salmonella or

Campylobacter infection *increases your risk for developing IBD by more than 100%.*[11]

"Dirty" Chickens

According to Consumer Reports, 8 out of 10 chickens harbor dangerous Salmonella and/or Campylobacter bacteria; these are the leading cause of foodborne illness. A total of 525 raw chickens were bought in stores nationwide and tested. The findings were shocking:

- 81% of chickens harbored Campylobacter
- 15% harbored Salmonella

This high level of bacterial contamination in chickens means that if you eat undercooked or poorly handled raw chicken, you can get very sick. Not only can you get fever, diarrhea, and abdominal cramps, but you are exposing yourself to a life-threatening neurological disease, Guillain-Barré syndrome (in case of exposure to Campylobacter bacteria).[12]

The Bottom Line:

Protect yourself against Salmonella or Campylobacter infections by taking these steps:

- Use a separate cutting board for meat and poultry.
- After handling chicken, sterilize your cutting board, knife, and sink area with hot, soapy water and bleach.
- Cook chicken soup for at least 1.5 hours or bake chicken until a meat thermometer shows an internal temperature of 165° F (75° C).

Antibiotic Resistance

Many of the contaminated chickens had antibiotic-resistant bacteria that:

"Showed resistance to one or more antibiotics, including some fed to chickens to speed their growth and those prescribed to humans to treat infections. The findings suggest that some people who are sickened by chicken might need to try several antibiotics before finding one that works."[13]

Contaminated Pre-cut Melons and Fruit Salad

In spring of 2019, The Centers for Disease Control and Prevention (CDC) issued a food safety alert. There was an outbreak of Salmonella infections, linked to pre-cut melons and fruit salad. 137 people from 10 states were infected. 38 people were hospitalized.[14]

The Bottom Line: Do not buy pre-cut fruit; buy whole fruit. Wash fruits well with soap and hot water, and dry with a paper towel prior to cutting. Refrigerate cut up fruit in dry, clean containers within 1 hour of cutting. This will minimize your chances of getting sick with salmonella.

Viruses and IBD Connection

Cytomegalovirus (CMV) infections may Trigger UC Flare

In ulcerative colitis, inflammation in the colon and long-term drug therapy with steroids and immunosuppressive can reactivate cytomegalovirus, which can make colon inflammation worse and exacerbate a UC flare.

According to French scientists' article published in the World Journal of Gastroenterology:

> *"CMV infection is frequent in ulcerative colitis (UC) and has been shown to be potentially harmful [...] Some treatments, notably steroids and cyclosporine A, have been shown to favor CMV reactivation, which seems not to be the case for therapies using anti-tumor necrosis factor drugs. According to these findings, in flare-ups of refractory UC, it is now recommended to look for the presence of CMV reactivation by using quantitative tools in colonic biopsies and to treat them with ganciclovir in cases of high viral load or severe disease."*[15]

Fungi and IBD Connection

The following scientific studies confirm that fungal overgrowth can be a key factor in the development of IBD.

Study #1: Fungal Overgrowth Results in Bowel Inflammation

Chinese scientists published a study where they analyzed 19 patients with active Crohn's disease. They compared the inflamed parts of the patients' gut lining (mucosa) to their non-inflamed gut lining. The study demonstrated that the inflamed mucosa had an overwhelming growth of 3 fungi: Candida albicans, Aspergillus clavatus, and Cryptococcus neoformans.

Researchers concluded: pathogenic fungal overgrowth results in bowel inflammation - a typical sign of IBD.[16]

Study #2: Fungus and Crohn's disease

In 2016, a team of international researchers from Case University School of Medicine identified "fungus as a key factor in the development of

Crohn's disease". In this study, researchers found that the fungus, Candida tropicalis, and two types of bacteria (E. coli and Serratia marcescens) form a slimy biofilm which sticks to the lining of the intestines, triggering gut inflammation and Crohn's disease symptoms. This study:

> *"Adds significant new information to understanding why some people develop Crohn's disease. Equally important, it can result in a new generation of treatments, including medications and probiotics, which hold the potential for making qualitative and quantitative differences in the lives of people suffering from Crohn's."*[17]

Study #3: Candida is the Most common Fungal Infection in IBD

It has been proven that patients with Crohn's disease and ulcerative colitis have an increased total fungal load in their intestinal mucosa and feces.

This is the result of intestinal yeast overgrowth, aka *candidiasis.*

The following symptoms of candidiasis can be painful and debilitating, especially for IBD people:

- Painful gas, bloating, and diarrhea
- Chronic fatigue, low energy, and depression
- Vaginal infections and urinary tract infections
- Persistent itching of skin, ears, rectum, and vagina

Balancing the fungal microbiota "can be considered as a therapeutic approach for IBD". This 2019 review article on fungal alterations in IBD was published in Alimentary Pharmacology & Therapeutics by scientists from Hong Kong, China.[18]

> *"Fourteen studies with data on 1524 patients were included in the final analysis. The most common fungal infections in patients with IBD were caused by Candida species (903 infections); the most commonly reported site of Candida infection was the gastrointestinal tract. Available evidence shows that most fungal infections occur within 12 months of IBD treatment and within 6 months when anti-TNFa agents are used."*[19]

Important Comment:

The saddest part of a debilitating disease like IBD is that many doctors don't understand that fungal overgrowth happens in many patients with Crohn's and ulcerative colitis. By treating a root cause like out-of-control fungal growth, it is very likely that many IBD patients will get better.

Based on my personal and clinical experience, and the research that I have done, I have incorporated anti-fungal foods and remedies into The Flare Stopper System.

Of course, IBD people must realize that exposure to antibiotics (via prescription drugs and foods), steroids, birth control pills, refined sugar, and alcohol is associated with disrupted balance of beneficial gut bacteria. This eventually leads to fungal overgrowth - one of the main causes of debilitating gut inflammation and intestinal lining injury in IBD.

Parasites and IBD Connection

E. histolytica causes Amebic Colitis and Crohn's disease

E. Histolytica (aka Entamoeba histolytica) is a common cause of infectious colitis and amebic abscess. The clinical, symptomatic, and endoscopic differentiation of amebic colitis and IBD is difficult, thereby increasing the likelihood of misdiagnoses. In many cases, amebic colitis is misdiagnosed as IBD, and is not diagnosed until surgery is needed. Symptoms in ulcerative colitis and amebic colitis are very similar: abdominal pain, bloody diarrhea, and weight loss.

Presence of Ameba detected in 35% of UC patients

In 2010, Turkish doctors from Research Hospital, Gastroenterology Department in Turkey, published a study in The European Journal of Internal Medicine on the presence of ameba parasites in patients with active ulcerative colitis. The results were shocking, because the rate of ameba infection was rather high. The study showed that out of 111 patients, amebiasis was detected in 35 (31.5%) patients.

> *"Stool samples were evaluated for presence of amebae using an Enzyme-Linked Immunosorbent Assay (ELISA) for detection of Entamoeba histolytica antigen."*

Study Conclusion:

> *"Any individual with ulcerative colitis who presents with symptoms of disease activation should be tested for ameba using antigen detection kits."*[20]

Also, Crohn's disease patients can suffer from ameba infections. Doctors from University Clinical Hospital Mostar in Bosnia discovered in their study that Crohn's disease group had 7 cases (20%) of E. histolytica infection out of 35 patients. Ulcerative colitis group had 12 cases (14.3%) of E. histolytica infection out of the 84 patients.

Control group who had no GI complaints, had only 2 cases (1.7%) of E. histolytica infection out of 119 patients.

Conclusion of the study:

> *"Ameba infections in patients with Crohn's disease and ulcerative colitis, have a greater prevalence compared to the normal population."*[21]

Treatment of Amebic Infection vs. Ulcerative Colitis

Doctors D. A. Shirley and S. Moonah from University of Virginia School of Medicine completed a scientific review of 24 patients with amebic colitis. Here are the distressing results:

- 58% were initially misdiagnosed with just colitis, then given steroids that resulted in rapid worsening of the disease
- Almost half of the patients had to have surgery
- 25% of patients died, despite receiving all the "appropriate" treatments with Flagyl[22]

Important Comment:

Your doctor, prior to prescribing corticosteroid drugs, MUST check your stool and blood for ameba infection. However, to make the whole case even more complicated, often patients' stool analysis for ameba presence can be negative. Out of multiple labs that checked my stool for Entamoeba histolytica, only one managed to find this parasite because this laboratory specialized in testing for gastrointestinal parasites.

So, if a patient is suspected of having an amebic infection, he must be treated with antibiotics and anti-parasitic medication. In such cases, the administration of steroid drugs should be avoided, because in cases of ameba infections, steroids work like adding gasoline to a fire. Believe me, I know - I almost died from this misdiagnosis (read my life story).

Giardia parasite can mimic Crohn's disease

Giardia lamblia is a microscopic parasite that lives in animal feces, human feces, contaminated food, water, and soil. The most common way for humans to get infected with Giardia is by drinking contaminated water, or swimming in lakes or swimming pools that contain Giardia. Other ways to get infected with Giardia is by exposure to feces infected with Giardia; you can be exposed by changing a sick child's diaper, not washing your hands, or through unprotected anal sex.

In their article *Crohn's disease and Infections*, Dr. Karel Geboes and Dr. Gert De Hertogh from University Hospital KU Leuven in Belgium talk about Giardia and Crohn's disease:

> *"Giardia lamblia infection of the small intestine can cause chronic abdominal pain, watery, foul-smelling stools associated with abdominal distension, anorexia, nausea, vomiting, weight loss, and malabsorption. Malabsorption can include steatorrhea, lactase deficiency, and malabsorption of fat-soluble vitamins and vitamin B12. The symptoms of chronic giardiasis can mimic Crohn's disease."*[23]

Correct Diagnosis is Vital

Based on the above, it is abundantly clear that correct diagnosis is vital in IBD management. Misdiagnoses can lead to severe worsening of the disease. Remember: tests must be done in specialized labs.

In the next chapter, you will learn about diagnosis and treatments of IBD.

References

[1] https://www.webmd.com/digestive-disorders/clostridium-difficile-colitis#1

[2] Sartor, R Balfour. "Mechanisms of disease: pathogenesis of Crohn's disease and ulcerative colitis." *Nature clinical practice. Gastroenterology & hepatology* vol. 3,7 (2006): 390-407. doi:10.1038/ncpgasthep0528

[3] Michael Greger, MD. "Paratuberculosis and Crohn's Disease: Got Milk?". January 2001

[4] Greenstein, Robert J. "Is Crohn's disease caused by a mycobacterium? Comparisons with leprosy, tuberculosis, and Johne's disease." *The Lancet. Infectious diseases* vol. 3,8 (2003): 507-14. doi:10.1016/s1473-3099(03)00724-2

[5] https://www.medicalnewstoday.com/articles/68511.php

[6] De Hertogh, Gert, and Karel Geboes. "Crohn's disease and infections: a complex relationship." *MedGenMed: Medscape general medicine* vol. 6,3 14. 10 Aug. 200

[7] https://www.medscape.com/viewarticle/540142_6

[8] https://www.livescience.com/64436-e-coli.html

[9] https://www.cdc.gov/campylobacter/index.html

[10] https://www.cdc.gov/salmonella/

[11] Dr. Nielsen et al. "Increased Short- and Long-Term Risk of Inflammatory Bowel Disease After Salmonella or Campylobacter Gastroenteritis". *Gastroenterology* 2009;137:495–501 https://www.gastrojournal.org/article/S0016-5085(09)00524-1/pdf

[12] https://www.consumerreports.org/media-room/press-releases/2007/01/consumer-reports-8-out-of-10-chickenstested-harbor-dangerous-bacteria/

[13] https://www.upc-online.org/health/120706consumerreports.html

[14] https://www.cdc.gov/salmonella/carrau-04-19/index.html

[15] Pillet, Sylvie et al. "Cytomegalovirus and ulcerative colitis: Place of antiviral therapy." *World journal of gastroenterology* vol. 22,6 (2016): 2030-45. doi:10.3748/wjg.v22.i6.2030 https://www.ncbi.nlm.nih.gov/pmc/articles/PMC4726676/

[16] Li, Qiurong et al. "Dysbiosis of gut fungal microbiota is associated with mucosal inflammation in Crohn's disease." *Journal of clinical gastroenterology* vol. 48,6 (2014): 513-23. doi:10.1097/MCG.0000000000000035
https://pubmed.ncbi.nlm.nih.gov/24275714/

[17] http://www.newswise.com/articles/case-western-reserve-led-international-team-identifies-fungus-in-humans-for-first-time-as-key-factor-in-crohn-s-disease

[18] Lam, Siu et al. "Review article: fungal alterations in inflammatory bowel diseases." *Alimentary pharmacology & therapeutics* vol. 50,11-12 (2019): 1159-1171. doi:10.1111/apt.15523
https://pubmed.ncbi.nlm.nih.gov/31648369/

[19] Stamatiades, George A et al. "Fungal infections in patients with inflammatory bowel disease: A systematic review." *Mycoses* vol. 61,6 (2018): 366-376. doi:10.1111/myc.12753
https://pubmed.ncbi.nlm.nih.gov/29453860/

[20] Ozin, Yasemin et al. "Presence and diagnosis of amebic infestation in Turkish patients with active ulcerative colitis." *European journal of internal medicine* vol. 20,5 (2009): 545-7. doi:10.1016/j.ejim.2009.05.014
https://pubmed.ncbi.nlm.nih.gov/19712863/

[21] Emil Babić et al. "Prevalence of amebiasis in inflammatory bowel disease in University Clinical Hospital Mostar". *Springerplus*. 2016; 5(1): 1586. Published online 2016 Sep 15. doi: 10.1186/s40064-016-3261-7

[22] Shirley, Debbie-Ann, and Shannon Moonah. "Fulminant Amebic Colitis after Corticosteroid Therapy: A Systematic Review." *PLoS neglected tropical diseases* vol. 10,7 e0004879. 28 Jul. 2016, doi:10.1371/journal.pntd.0004879
https://pubmed.ncbi.nlm.nih.gov/27467600/

[23] De Hertogh, Gert, and Karel Geboes. "Crohn's disease and infections: a complex relationship." *MedGenMed: Medscape general medicine* vol. 6,3 14. 10 Aug. 2004

CHAPTER 5

Proper tests and diagnosis are vital for effective treatment of IBD

How do you figure out if you have a disease?

YOU GO TO A MEDICAL PROFESSIONAL WHO LEARNS ABOUT YOUR medical history and health issues. The medical professional then applies techniques like physical examination, lab work, and different types of tests.

Using all the information gathered, the medical professional establishes a diagnosis identifying a disease or condition in you. This diagnosis then implies what treatments are necessary.

Are diagnoses always correct?

Sometimes, even medical professionals get things wrong. They can be incorrect about what disease or condition you have. This is called a misdiagnosis. A misdiagnosis can lead to wrong treatments.

Misdiagnosis and the consequential wrong treatment are dangerous, and can lead to disastrous results.

I experienced misdiagnosis firsthand, and it led to more than a year of needless suffering. So, I dedicated decades of my professional life to this subject.

When I first got sick, doctors misdiagnosed me with ulcerative colitis. They tested me for parasites & bacteria using my stool sample. Every time, the results came back negative, so they diagnosed me with ulcerative colitis. It turns out, the tests were inaccurate, and I had an amoebic infection.

The symptoms of ulcerative colitis and amoebic colitis are identical: bloody diarrhea with mucus, abdominal pain, severe weight loss, and dehydration. During amoebic colitis, introduction of steroids works like putting gasoline on fire. The amoeba parasite becomes more aggressive and invasive resulting in marked deterioration of patients' symptoms. That is why my condition got worse. Don't ever give steroids to people with amoeba infection, because it can lead to deadly fulminant amoebic colitis. I was put on this treatment for more than a year.

Why Does Misdiagnosis Happen in IBD?

Misdiagnosis in IBD is common, because:

1. Symptoms of bacterial/parasitic infections are similar to symptoms of IBD.
2. Testing of some bacterial/parasitic infections is notoriously inadequate.
3. Even when diagnosed correctly, the treatment itself can trigger more infections with different pathogens and/or cause the same symptoms as a patient experiencing a flare.

I'll explain why in a minute. Believe me, I know - I was one of such misdiagnosed patients. This misdiagnosis with the following wrong treatment almost killed me. You can read more about it in the chapter "My Life Story".

Getting Correct Diagnoses is Vital for Properly Treating IBD

Correct diagnosis of ulcerative colitis is NOT AT ALL a straightforward task for your doctors. Quite the contrary. The fact is ulcerative colitis and bacterial/parasitic infection have very similar symptoms - but they are two very different medical conditions. Wrong diagnosis leads to wrong treatment which, if not corrected, can be DEADLY.

Bacterial infections caused by invasive bacteria (e.g., C. difficile), or parasitic infections (e.g., amoeba like E. histolytica) can mimic ulcerative colitis.

Stephen Hanauer, MD discussed this problem recently in Medscape Gastroenterology. He suggested that a physician should rule out possible mimics of ulcerative colitis before confirming diagnoses.[1]

IBD can resemble other diseases

The Japanese Society of Gastroenterology states in their Guidelines for IBD:

> *"It is often necessary to distinguish UC from infectious enterocolitis, especially Campylobacter, invasive Escherichia coli, and amoebic dysentery. Excluding these diseases by bacteriological and parasitological examinations is indispensable to make a diagnosis of UC. The symptoms of the acute stage of CD may resemble those of acute appendicitis or colonic diverticulitis, and it may be difficult to differentiate intestinal tuberculosis or intestinal Behçet's disease from CD before the final diagnosis of CD is established."*[2]

The Bottom Line: To properly determine what type of infection a patient might have; the doctor needs to order various tests. Only based on the results of such tests would a physician be able to select a proper treatment option.

Look for doctors trained in treatment of parasitic and bacterial infections. They usually specialize in Tropical Medicine, and are called infectious disease specialists. It is highly recommended to rule out any GI infection prior to starting The Flare Stopper System.

Next, let's discover which pathogens are especially hard to diagnose.

Parasitic Infections

IBD and parasitic infections have many symptoms in common, such as bloody diarrhea, abdominal pain, GI inflammation and ulcerations.

Parasitic infections may be caused by the following:

- Eating contaminated food
- Drinking contaminated water that was not boiled
- Swallowing contaminated lake/river water while swimming
- Touching surfaces contaminated by an infected person: diapers, bathroom fixtures, etc.
- Sexual contact [3]

The most common parasitic infections in the gut are from the following parasites: Giardia, Cryptosporidium, and Entamoeba histolytica.

Diagnoses

Unfortunately, some doctors still use a simple stool test as the main indicator for parasitic infections. This test is called ova and parasites (O&P). In this test, your stool sample is examined under a microscope by a lab technician, who looks for parasites and their eggs (ova) shedding from your large intestine into your stool. The truth is - this test is grossly inadequate.

This test is especially inadequate for the Entamoeba histolytica intestinal parasite. According to the World Health Organization (WHO), this parasite infects approximately 50 million people and causes 100,000 deaths annually, worldwide. These people can get sick with colitis and develop liver abscesses.[4]

Entamoeba histolytica

I was one of those infected with Entamoeba histolytica. If you read my story chapter, you can recall the misdiagnosis of my amoebic colitis due to negative stool test results from different labs.

Why is misdiagnosis so common?

Here is my explanation:

1. To detect a parasite, especially E. histolytica, at least 3 stool samples must be examined within 10 days because "these organisms may be excreted intermittently or may be unevenly distributed in the stool."

   These findings were presented in a scientific article "Laboratory Diagnostic Techniques for Entamoeba Species" published in Clinical Microbiology Reviews in 2007.[5]

   The need for multiple stool samples also has been confirmed by Dr. Amin, the founder of Parasitology Center in Tempe, Arizona. Here is his opinion:

   "Entamoeba histolytica is active for one or two days, and then is not typically active or detectable the next day or two." This means that if "the stool sample is collected

from a patient with one of these cyclical parasites on a day when the pathogen is not active, it won't be in the stool and obviously won't be detected by testing. However, this doesn't mean that there's no infection present."[6]

2. Ideally, a stool test should be done within 1 hour after the stool sample is passed by the patient, otherwise, E. Histolytica degrades rapidly.[5]

   In real life, it takes many hours between a patient producing a stool sample and a lab technician examining it, making detection almost impossible.

3. Diagnosis of pathogenic E. histolytica is difficult. Here is why: some pathogenic amoebae look very similar to non-pathogenic amoebae. For example, Entamoeba histolytica is a pathogenic organism. It causes amoebiasis, which produces diarrhea with or without blood. Entamoeba histolytica looks very similar to Entamoeba Dispar, a non-pathogenic organism that can live in your gut without making you sick.

When your stool sample is examined under a microscope, lab technicians can have a hard time differentiating between these pathogenic and non-pathogenic types of amoebae. Misdiagnosis is the result.

According to scientists from Stanford University, examination of stool for ova and parasite misses from 50% to 75% of all E. histolytica infections detected by more accurate tests.[7]

How to Accurately Diagnose E. Histolytica

Your doctor can order a new alternative in addition to the simple O&P test. This new test is a monoclonal antibody-based ELISA (Enzyme Linked Immunosorbent Immunoassay), specifically designed to detect E. Histolytica. The test is performed by Tech Lab. This type of test is recommended by the World Health Organization (WHO).[7, 5]

Find links to these testing facilities at http://knowyourgut.com/resources/

If the first and second tests come back negative, make sure your doctor orders at least three stool sample tests over a 10-day period.

Ensure that your stool sample is examined within 60 minutes of you passing the stool.

If the parasite has not been found in your stool and your symptoms persist, then another test should be done using your blood. This test is called E. Histolytica antibody (IgG), ELISA. Your immune system makes antibodies when it fights an infection like E. Histolytica. This test does have one limitation: in some cases, the presence of antibodies shows past exposure to this parasite (not a current infection).

The PCI Parasitology Center is a lab that is popular with doctors practicing alternative medicine and with those interested in various GI infections, especially parasites. This lab is managed by Dr. Omar Amin, who has published dozens of scientific research articles in the field of parasitology and infectious diseases.

Physicians who use this lab claim that Dr. Amin can detect parasites and infections in patients whose results came back negative from other labs.

Find links to parasite testing facilities at
http://knowyourgut.com/resources/

E. Histolytica Treatment

If a patient is suspected of having amoebic infection, they are usually treated with antibiotics (like metronidazole) and anti-parasitic medication (like diloxanide furoate or iodoquinol).

In case of amoeba infection, steroid drugs should be avoided. Adding steroids to an amoeba infection is like adding gasoline to a fire. It can result in rapid progression of IBD leading to surgeries and in some cases, death.

In severe cases of amoebic dysentery, tetracycline antibiotics are prescribed (e.g., doxycycline).[8]

Giardia and Cryptosporidium

Giardia and Cryptosporidium Diagnosis

One of the best tests for Giardia and Cryptosporidium detection is done by Meridian Bioscience. The test is called Merifluor™ Cryptosporidium/ Giardia.[9]

Find the link here: http://knowyourgut.com/resources/

The Center for Disease Control and Prevention (CDC) has tons of very useful information about transmission, detection (diagnoses), and treatments of parasitic diseases, find the link here: http://knowyourgut.com/resources/

Giardia Treatment

According to Mayo Clinic, patients with persistent, severe giardia infections are treated with the following medications:

- **Flagyl (Metronidazole)** is a popular antibiotic for parasitic infections including giardia.
- **Tindamax (Tinidazole)** is an antibiotic that is used to treat parasitic infections.
- **Alinia (Nitazoxanide)** - is broad-spectrum antiparasitic and antiviral medication.[10]

Cryptosporidium Treatment

According to the CDC, "immunocompromised patients may have more severe complications, such as life-threatening malabsorption and wasting. Diarrheal illness may be accompanied by fever or fatigue."[11]

That is why treatment of cryptosporidium for immunocompromised patients includes three types of medications:

- **Anti-parasitic:** Alinia (Nitazoxanide) attacks the parasite.
- **Antibiotic:** Azithromycin (Zithromax) is used to prevent opportunistic infections in immunocompromised patients.
- **Antidiarrheal:** Imodium A-D relieves diarrhea by increasing fluid absorption in the intestines. It decreases the number of daily bowel movements and makes your stool less watery.[12]

Bacterial Infections

Bacterial gastrointestinal infections are often caused by food poisoning after eating undercooked beef, poultry, eggs, or milk. The infections can also come from drinking water contaminated with pathogenic bacteria such as Salmonella, Campylobacter, and E. coli. In patients taking antibiotics, the bacterium Clostridium difficile can cause life-threatening colon inflammation and watery diarrhea (sometimes with blood).

Clostridium Difficile

Clostridium Difficile infection is a serious health threat. According to the CDC, almost half a million people get sick with C. diff in the United States annually. "One in 11 people over age 65 diagnosed with a healthcare-associated C. diff infection die within one month."[13]

Even more disturbing: an increasing number of patients are diagnosed with severe C. difficile colitis. In these patients, early detection of C. diff infection is crucial for preserving the patient's life.[14]

An accurate diagnosis of C. diff infection (CDI) can be difficult.

To date, "there is no single stool test that can be relied upon as the reference standard for the diagnosis of CDI." This opinion was stated by multiple doctors from the US and China in a review article published in Emerging Microbes & Infections.[14]

Moreover, some people can carry C. diff while not getting sick from it. They are C. diff carriers, but their diarrhea is caused by something else.[15]

Because of the above diagnostic difficulties, doctors should use algorithmic testing, which requires clinical assessment of patients' symptoms, and doing multiple tests to confirm CDI. Also, the doctor should ask whether the patient was taking antibiotics in the last 3 months.

ATTENTION:

1. IBD patients who take antibiotics (e.g., Cipro, Levaquin), immunosuppressants (e.g. methotrexate), and proton pump inhibitors (e.g. Prevacid) are at increased risk of developing serious colon infection from Clostridium Difficile (C. diff).[16]
2. Also, IBD patients should be aware that use of steroids in IBD is "associated with threefold increase in developing C. diff". Therefore, decrease in steroids is recommended, especially in hospitalized IBD patients.[17]
3. Patients with an ileo-anal pouch should know that they are at high risk of developing C. difficile infection. So, if you have an ileo-anal pouch and are experiencing an increase in daily stools and weight loss, your doctor should test you for C. diff infection.[18]

How to Accurately Diagnose Clostridium Difficile Infection

Only liquid stool specimens (diarrhea-type) should be processed by the laboratory. The stool specimens should be cultured within 2 hours after collection.

A doctor should use algorithmic testing to first identify if a patient is a "C. diff carrier". For that they need to order Nucleic Acid Amplification

Testing (NAAT), which confirms the presence of the C. difficile toxin gene.

Because the NAAT test detects the toxin gene and not the toxins produced by C. diff bacteria, NAAT should be followed by a Toxin A & B test. This test confirms if a patient has an active C. diff infection.

FYI, when C. diff starts to grow, it produces toxins A and B, causing diarrhea and colitis. So, when a patient has an active C. diff infection, toxin A and/or B are present in the patient's stool.[19]

If the toxin A/B test is positive, C. diff infection is present, and must be treated ASAP.

Treatment

Oral vancomycin antibiotic is recommended for eradication of C. diff infection. The duration and dosage of vancomycin are determined by your physician.

The antibiotic metronidazole is *not* recommended due to poor response - its failure rate is about 50%.[17]

Escherichia coli (E. coli) and Campylobacter

E. coli bacteria is a part of healthy intestinal flora. But a pathogenic strain, such as E. coli O157:H7 can cause vomiting, bloody diarrhea, and cramps. You can get infected with E. coli from eating undercooked ground beef and raw vegetables contaminated with E. coli.[20]

According to the CDC, campylobacter causes an estimated 1.5 million illnesses each year in the United States.[21]

The main sources of campylobacter infection are: undercooked meat, raw or contaminated milk, contaminated water, and ice. You can kill Campylobacter bacteria by cooking food thoroughly, and boiling water and milk. Avoid drinking beverages with ice made from unfiltered, non-boiled water.

Diagnosis of E. coli and Campylobacter

Stool antigen detection tests are some of the best methods to detect foodborne pathogenic bacteria (Shiga toxin-producing E. coli and Campylobacter). I've listed the best ones here: http://knowyourgut.com/resources/

Share with your doctor.

Treatment of E. coli

According to the Cleveland Clinic, if you have E. coli infection, you should not take antibiotics and/or medications that stop diarrhea (such as Imodium) because that will make the E. coli infection worse. It will also increase your risk of a deadly form of kidney failure, called hemolytic uremic syndrome (HUS). There is no medication that can cure E. coli infection. Rest and drink at least 2.5 liters (about 10 cups) of fluid every 24 hours.[22]

Treatment for Campylobacter

Uncomplicated cases do not require medical treatment. Patients with invasive infection with bloody diarrhea and a high fever are usually treated with one of the following antibiotics: azithromycin, erythromycin, or clarithromycin.

Salmonella

According to The Center for Disease Control and Prevention (CDC), Salmonella bacteria causes about 1.3 million infections in the US every year. Salmonella bacterial infection is also known as salmonellosis, or acute gastroenteritis.

One can get sick after eating contaminated sausages, pork, beef, chicken, or drinking contaminated water. Also, contact with infected animal feces (e.g., from chickens, birds, or reptiles) can result in Salmonella infection or gastroenteritis. So, remember to wash your hands with hot water and soap for at least 20 seconds after handling animals and birds.

Diagnosis of Salmonella

These tests are used to diagnose salmonella infection:

1. Fresh stool test
2. Blood culture

Treatment of Salmonella

If a patient has uncomplicated Salmonella gastroenteritis, antibiotics are not recommended. However, a short, 3–5-day course of Ceftriaxone therapy is indicated in the following cases: immunocompromised patients, patients with severe colitis, and patients with invasive Salmonella infection. Doctors from Chang Gung Memorial Hospital in Chiayi, Taiwan say:

> *"Antibiotics should be discontinued as soon as possible when the patient's clinical condition improves."*[23]

Other antibiotics are also used, depending on patients' condition and the results of in vitro susceptibility testing. This is where the salmonella pathogen is isolated from the patient's specimen, then tested against several antibiotics. This test helps identify the appropriate antibiotic treatment of the particular Salmonella strain. Not all antibiotics work against all Salmonella strains.

Fungal Infections

Numerous studies have confirmed that patients with ulcerative colitis and Crohn's disease have persistent fungal/yeast infection in their gut.

Diagnoses

A comprehensive DNA stool test called GI-MAP can identify if you have fungal overgrowth in your gut. It is offered by the Diagnostic Solutions laboratory. A GI-MAP test can also be very useful in determining the level of inflammation in the gut, and potential bacterial autoimmune triggers. Find the test here: http://knowyourgut.com/resources/

If you don't have the money to do the GI-MAP test, and you want to re-establish healthy gut flora, consider addressing fungal overgrowth as part of your gut restoration program. The book you are holding right now can help you do just that.

Treatment

More than 25 years ago, I realized that getting rid of fungal/yeast infection must be an integral part of a gut restoration program, especially during a flare. This concept has been recently confirmed by scientists from Hong Kong, China. Their study stated that balancing the fungal microbiota "can be considered as a therapeutic approach for IBD." The study was published in Alimentary Pharmacology & Therapeutics.[24]

Some functional medicine doctors use antifungal drug Nystatin and/or Fluconazole to treat gastrointestinal candidiasis and other fungal infections. Be aware that these drugs can cause nausea, vomiting, and diarrhea.

Therefore, unless a patient has a severe case of fungal/yeast infection, I prefer to use natural methods for getting rid of fungal issues. Severe cases must be determined by a doctor.

The Conclusion

After the pathogens have been identified and treated as needed, you can start The Flare Stopper System.

In essence, your goal should be to create a healthy biological terrain in your gut that can fight off pathogens easily. We are all exposed to pathogens, but it's the strength of our microbiome that determines whether we get sick from them.

A strong microbiome can be nurtured via a gut-healing diet, detoxification, and the right mindset...let's do it.

In the next chapter, we'll review conventional treatments for IBD.

References

[1] Stephen Hanauer, MD. "The 5 Goals of Colonoscopy in Ulcerative Colitis." *Medscape Gastroenterology* - May 21, 2021.
https://www.medscape.com/viewarticle/950489

[2] Matsuoka, Katsuyoshi et al. "Evidence-based clinical practice guidelines for inflammatory bowel disease." *Journal of gastroenterology* vol. 53,3 (2018): 305-353. doi:10.1007/s00535-018-1439-1
https://www.ncbi.nlm.nih.gov/pmc/articles/PMC5847182/

[3] https://www.cdc.gov/parasites/crypto/infection-sources.html

[4] Tanyuksel, Mehmet, and William A Petri Jr. "Laboratory diagnosis of amebiasis." *Clinical microbiology reviews* vol. 16,4 (2003): 713-29. doi:10.1128/CMR.16.4.713-729.2003

[5] R. Fotedar, et al. "Laboratory Diagnostic Techniques for Entamoeba Species." *Clinical Microbiology Reviews* Jul 2007, 20 (3) 511-532; DOI: 10.1128/CMR.00004-07

[6] Nancy Faass and Trent Nichols, MD, *Optimal Digestive Wellness*, pg. 134. Healing Arts Press, 1999

[7] William A. Petri, Jr., Upinder Singh, "Diagnosis and Management of Amebiasis". *Clinical Infectious Diseases*, Volume 29, Issue 5, November 1999, Pages 1117–1125, https://doi.org/10.1086/313493

[8] https://iliveok.com/health/treatment-amebiasis-drugs_110983i15955.html

[9] Johnston, Stephanie P et al. "Evaluation of three commercial assays for detection of Giardia and Cryptosporidium organisms in fecal specimens." *Journal of clinical microbiology* vol. 41,2 (2003): 623-6. doi:10.1128/JCM.41.2.623-626.2003

[10] https://www.mayoclinic.org/diseases-conditions/giardia-infection/diagnosis-treatment/drc-20372790

[11] https://www.cdc.gov/dpdx/cryptosporidiosis/index.html

[12] https://www.mayoclinic.org/diseases-conditions/cryptosporidium/diagnosis-treatment/drc-20351876

[13] https://www.cdc.gov/cdiff/what-is.html

[14] https://www.ncbi.nlm.nih.gov/pmc/articles/PMC5837143/

[15] Putting C. Difficile to the Test by Abbott https://www.globalpointofcare.abbott/en/knowledge-insights/stories/putting-c-diff-to-test-us.html

[16] C Gateau et al. "How to: diagnose infection caused by Clostridium difficile" *CMI Clinical Microbiology and Infection*. Volume 24, issue 5, P463-468, May 01, 2018 https://www.clinicalmicrobiologyandinfection.com/article/S1198-743X(17)30678-X/fulltext

[17] https://www.med.unc.edu/gi/ibd/files/2018/05/Clostridium_diff_and_IBD.pdf

[18] Li, Yue et al. "Risk factors and outcome of PCR-detected Clostridium difficile infection in ileal pouch patients." *Inflammatory bowel diseases* vol. 19,2 (2013): 397-403. doi:10.1097/MIB.0b013e318280fcb9

[19] https://labtestsonline.org/tests/clostridium-difficile-and-c-diff-toxin-testing

[20] https://www.mayoclinic.org/diseases-conditions/e-coli/symptoms-causes/syc-20372058

[21] https://www.cdc.gov/campylobacter/index.html

[22] https://my.clevelandclinic.org/health/diseases/16638-e-coli-infection/management-and-treatment

[23] Chen, Hung-Ming et al. "Nontyphoid salmonella infection: microbiology, clinical features, and antimicrobial therapy." *Pediatrics and neonatology* vol. 54,3 (2013): 147-52. doi:10.1016/j.pedneo.2013.01.010
https://www.sciencedirect.com/science/article/pii/S1875957213000119

[24] Lam, Siu et al. "Review article: fungal alterations in inflammatory bowel diseases." *Alimentary pharmacology & therapeutics* vol. 50,11-12 (2019): 1159-1171. doi:10.1111/apt.15523
https://pubmed.ncbi.nlm.nih.gov/31648369/

CHAPTER 6

Conventional Treatments of IBD

Usually, GI doctors only offer 3 ways to manage IBD:

1. Drugs
2. Surgery
3. Both: Drugs and surgery

My own doctors said, "IBD drugs can induce and maintain remission" ... Is that true?

My doctors tried to treat my ulcerative colitis with medication for 10 years. After all those years of treatment with medications, I eventually stopped responding to all prescription drugs.

My diarrhea, bleeding, and malnutrition continued despite of all my prescribed steroids, anti-inflammatories, antibiotics, and anti-parasitic medications. And I was offered what my doctors called the ultimate cure - surgery (colectomy).

Don't get me wrong - I am not against medications. Medications can be effective for a short time and may be needed to arrest a flare. However, long-term use of medications is often ineffective, and can cause serious side effects. Most importantly, these IBD drugs do not address the root cause of the IBD problem.

Like me, many colitis and Crohn's patients are disappointed and frustrated with the conventional medical treatments offered to them. For years, these patients have been told by their doctors, "The cause of UC and CD is unknown. These conditions cannot be cured; you can only manage it with drugs and surgeries."

Should you take prescription drugs for life?

The gastroenterologists are saying that you MUST take prescription drugs FOR LIFE in order to achieve and maintain remission. On paper, it sounds great. However, in real life, long-term usage of drugs just does not work. Even in a best-case scenario, these drugs suppress disease symptoms temporarily, while the root causes of IBD are ignored.

As years go by, the IBD patient is prescribed more prescription drugs to control the disease - but the exhausted IBD patient just gets sicker.

They start losing hope for normal, healthy living because the disease gets out of control and starts to affect other organs as well (joints, eyes, liver, pancreas, endocrine system). In addition, patients often experience severe side effects from medications, ranging from bloody diarrhea, nausea, and vomiting to a suppressed immune system, serious infections, pancreatitis, hepatitis, and even cancer.

The Conclusion

Medications, especially taken long-term, cannot cure IBD. These drugs are designed to suppress or inhibit healthy bodily functions.

While some IBD drugs can temporarily improve your symptoms and bring you much needed remission, when taken long-term, they weaken your immune system, damage your organs, and further exacerbate gut inflammation. That is the reason why so many sick IBD people just get sicker and cannot get better.

This is not just my opinion.

According to Dr. Chang-Tai Xu from 4th Military Medical University in China:

"There is no medication that can cure Ulcerative Colitis."

Dr. Chang-Tai Xu and his team expressed this opinion in a 2004 article called "Drug therapy for ulcerative colitis" (published in the prestigious World Journal of Gastroenterology).[1]

Let's take a closer look at the efficacy of drugs and surgery:

Treatment #1 - Drugs

First, let's look at drugs as a treatment. There are 5 types of drugs used in IBD (Colitis and Crohn's):

1. Aminosalicylates (aka 5-ASAs)
2. Steroids (aka Corticosteroids)
3. Immunosuppressants
4. Biologics
5. Antibiotics

Also, some medications have two names: the generic name and the brand name. For example, the steroid medication Uceris (brand name) is also known as Budesonide (generic name).

Let's learn about each drug type, examples, drawbacks, and side effects.

1. Aminosalicylates

What are they & how do they work?

Aminosalicylates are anti-inflammatory drugs prescribed to IBD patients to treat intestinal inflammation and to prevent flare-ups. The active ingredient in aminosalicylate is called 5-aminosalicylic acid (5-ASA for short).

Aminosalicylates work by decreasing the production of inflammatory chemicals (aka prostaglandins) in the mucous lining of the colon. Doctors usually prescribe aminosalicylates to newly diagnosed patients with mild to moderate ulcerative colitis and mild forms of Crohn's disease. IBD patients can take aminosalicylates by mouth (via tablet or capsules) or rectally (via enema, rectal foams, or suppositories.)

Examples

Some examples of aminosalicylates are:

- Azulfidine
- Apriso
- Canasa
- Pentasa
- Rowasa
- Lialda
- Delzicol
- Salofalk
- Colazal
- Giazo
- Dipentum

Drawbacks

Here is what Sherry A. Rogers, MD says about sulfasalazine in her popular book *No More Heartburn*:

> *"Sulfasalazine, also known by the trade name Azulfidine and (its new cousin) Asacol, is a time-honored drug. Side effects include kidney or lung damage so severe it can be lethal, paralysis (Guillain-Barre syndrome), hepatitis, depression, vision problems, and even a low white blood cell count (leukopenia) and a decreased level of blood clotting cells (thrombocytopenia), both of which are particularly dangerous for someone already rundown by intestinal infection and bleeding. Sulfasalazine is universally prescribed for most colitis patients, in the acute stage as well as "forever" with hopes of keeping them in remission. It is a glorified aspirin (NSAID) and sulfa drug rolled into one. By now you recognize that as a deadly duo guaranteed to make and maintain a leaky gut indefinitely. And that is one reason colitis patients rarely recover permanently. They are prescribed drugs that perpetuate the disease and, in fact, worsen it, methodically decreasing the chance for recovery."*[2]

You might think this is just the opinion of one doctor.

Well, let's see what possible side effects Pfizer (the manufacturer of this drug) lists in their drug insert for Azulfidine:

> *"Hepatitis, hepatic failure, pancreatitis, bloody diarrhea, impaired folic acid absorption, impaired digoxin absorption, stomatitis, diarrhea, abdominal pains, and neutropenic enterocolitis."*[3]

Azulfidine can also cause male infertility (reduced sperm count) as well as malabsorption of folate B vitamin, folate, which is required for healthy cell growth and function.

In the late 1980's, when I learned that the Azulfidine (sulfasalazine) I was taking could cause bloody diarrhea and abdominal pain, I started to wonder... Do I have bloody diarrhea and abdominal pain from colitis? Or is it from this medication?

Think about it. You are taking a medication that is supposed to lower gut inflammation and stop your bleeding and diarrhea. But the very same medication can also *cause* bloody diarrhea and abdominal pain. How does that make sense? That's what I thought when taking Azulfidine. So - I stopped taking it.

I bled *before* taking Azulfidine. I bled *while* taking it. And I bled *after* stopping it. It didn't make any difference for me.

Also, according to The Japanese Society of Gastroenterology guidelines for IBD, 5-ASA fails to maintain remission in Crohn's disease:

> *"The lack of efficacy of 5-ASA for maintenance of remission in CD is confirmed by the meta-analysis of placebo-controlled trials with a sufficient sample size"*[4]

Side effects

The most common side effects of aminosalicylates are: diarrhea, nausea, fever, rash, headache, and reduced sperm count in men.

What happens if aminosalicylates fail

As you can see from the Japanese study above, aminosalicylates may not be as effective as one would hope for keeping Crohn's patients in remission. For some patients, it takes time to understand these drugs are not working. These "unresponsive" patients are then offered something else: steroids.

Let's examine the efficacy of steroids.

2. Steroids (aka Corticosteroids)

What are they & how do they work?

Steroids are prescribed to IBD patients who are not responding to aminosalicylates. Steroids are used to reduce immune system activity and to lower inflammation in the digestive tract.

My Story about Steroids

After aminosalicylates failed for me, my GI doctor prescribed me steroids - 40mg of prednisone daily.

I was in a flare, and after taking the prednisone, I noticed significant improvement to my symptoms in less than a week (less bloody diarrhea, no abdominal pain).

Once my flare subsided, the prednisone dose was reduced gradually by 5mg per week, until I fully discontinued prednisone...until my next flare.

And so, this pattern repeated. I'd have a flare, take steroids, the flare would go away… and then the flare would come back. And I'd be prescribed yet another round of steroids.

The first few years I was on prednisone cycles, it worked like a charm in stopping my UC flares - the first couple of times. However, over time, I became dependent on these steroids.

I would suffer from flares whenever my steroid dose dropped below 20mg.

In addition to UC flares, my long-term steroid use resulted in the loss of my bone density. I was eventually diagnosed with osteoporosis. It turns out that steroids can cause osteoporosis by increasing calcium loss in kidneys and bones, while decreasing calcium absorption from intestines.

Furthermore, while taking steroids, I suffered from depression, insomnia, moon face (facial swelling), and frequent infections. Later, I learned that my experience was not unique; many IBD patients experience similar side effects. In my case, many years ago, when those side effects took a great toll on me, my doctor recommended I stop taking steroids gradually.

Steroids are similar to the hormone cortisol, which is produced by your adrenal glands. In addition to their anti-inflammatory work, steroids trick your body into thinking it has produced enough cortisol, and therefore your glands' natural cortisol production is either greatly reduced or shut down completely.

When you take steroids, your adrenal glands get the message to reduce or stop cortisol production. So, if you've been taking steroid drugs, and suddenly stop, your adrenal glands are not able to respond quickly enough with their own steroid production. This results in adrenal insufficiency.

This adrenal insufficiency causes a great deal of stress on your body which can result in fatigue, nausea, vomiting, fever, and another flare.

Taper steroids slowly - NEVER DISCONTINUE STEROIDS ABRUPTLY. You can experience adrenal insufficiency. Consult your physician on a tapering schedule.

Drawbacks

Steroids fail to keep patients in remission. My disastrous experience with steroids was finally validated in 2016, by clinical practice guidelines issued by The Japanese Society of Gastroenterology for the treatment of ulcerative colitis and Crohn's disease.

Here's what their guidelines say:

> *"Corticosteroids have no efficacy for maintenance of remission. Long-term or high-dose use of steroids should be avoided and they should not be used to maintain remission because of their various side effects such as immunosuppression, impaired glucose tolerance, a delay in wound healing, and osteoporosis."*[4]

Finally, doctors are realizing the simple truth that I and many others experienced over 25 years ago: *long-term steroid treatment simply does not work.*

Examples

Depending on the location of your IBD, different types of steroidal drugs are used. Here are some examples:

- Oral steroids: Deltasone, Prednisolone, Medrol, Hydrocortisone, Uceris, Entocort EC
- Rectal steroids (in the form of foams/suppositories/enemas): Cortenema, Medrol, Anucort-HC, Anusol-HC, ProctoFoam-HC

Side effects

The CDC (Center for Disease Control) warns that steroids can weaken the immune system when taken long-term, resulting in serious fungal infections.[5]

See the CDC's list of oral corticosteroids below that can increase the chances of getting a fungal infection.

- Budesonide (Entocort EC)
- Cortisone (Cortone)
- Dexamethasone (Decadron)
- Hydrocortisone (Cortef)
- Methylprednisolone (Medrol)

- Prednisolone (Prelone)
- Prednisone (Deltasone)
- Triamcinolone

Here is the CDC's list of serious fungal infections:

- Histoplasmosis
- Cryptococcosis
- Coccidioidomycosis
- Invasive Candida infection
- Pneumocystis pneumonia
- Invasive aspergillosis

Used long-term, steroids cause muscle wasting, increased risk of infection, and interference with calcium absorption, resulting in brittle bones. That is why many patients are forced to stop steroid treatments.

The problems with steroids were discussed in a scientific review published in Gastroenterology journal:

> *"Corticosteroids are limited in their use by risk of infection, osteoporosis, hypertension, growth retardation, poor mucosal healing, and early relapses on cessation of therapy. This is especially problematic in paediatric patients who may experience significant growth retardation and osteoporosis with steroid therapy."*[6]

What happens if steroids fail

When treatments with aminosalicylates and steroids fail to control the intestinal inflammation, or when a patient cannot quit steroids without causing another flare, doctors prescribe immunosuppressant medications. Their line of thinking is that Crohn's disease and ulcerative colitis are autoimmune diseases, which are driven by an overactive immune response.

So, instead of addressing disbalance in gut microbiota, the patient's own immunity is suppressed with immunosuppressant drugs, in an attempt to induce remission.

3. Immunosuppressants

What are they & how do they work?

Immunosuppressants are prescribed to IBD patients who are not responding to aminosalicylates and steroids. Immunosuppressants, as you might expect from the name, suppress the immune system. They are used to lower the level of inflammation in IBD by weakening the body's immune response.

Examples

Examples of immunosuppressants include:

- 6-Mercaptopurine (6-MP, Purinethol)
- Methotrexate
- Azathioprine (Imuran)
- Cyclosporine (Sandimmune)

Drawbacks

Because these drugs suppress the immune system, they disable your body's ability to fight against infections and pathogens. This increases your risk of infection. According to a 2017 review article published in Pharmaceutical Journal, when using immunosuppressants, it may take up to 6 months for these drugs to start working. "So, these agents are not useful for induction of remission."[7]

Side effects

Immunosuppressants can cause worsening of diarrhea, flu-like illness with fever, body aches and pains, anemia, reduced kidney function, inflammation of pancreas, liver cirrhosis, and increased risk of cancer. While taking immunosuppressants, make sure you have regular blood tests to monitor your kidney and liver function.

What happens if immunosuppressants fail

When treatments with immunosuppressants fail to control IBD flares, doctors prescribe biologics.

4. Biologics

What are they & how do they work?

If you do not respond to the above treatments, doctors will prescribe biologics, also known as TNF (tumor necrosis factor) inhibitors. They are also called anti-TNF drugs, or TNF blockers.

Our bodies naturally produce TNF-alpha protein as part of our immune response. When IBD patients experience chronic intestinal inflammation, they have elevated levels of TNF-alpha. The biologics (aka TNF inhibitors) bind to this TNF-alpha and block its release from the cells. After taking biologics, some patients experience reduction in symptoms and intestinal inflammation. It can take at least 2 months to see improvement in symptoms - however, biologics do not work for every IBD patient.

Examples

Examples of biologics include:

- Infliximab (Remicade)

- Adalimumab (Humira)
- Golimumab (Simponi)
- Certolizumab (Cimzia)
- Etanercept (Enbrel)

Drawbacks

1. **Biologics are very expensive.**

   In 2015, biologic drug cost per adult patient, per year, was $36,051. The cost for a child patient was even higher, at $41,109 per year. Although many insurance plans do cover biologic drugs, IBD patients still often spend a lot of money in co-pay fees.[8]

2. **Many IBD patients fail to achieve remission with biologics.**

   Also, only 45% of Crohn's patients respond to treatments with biologics. So, 55% of patients (*over half*), do not respond to biologics. "Studies also indicate that 50-70% of all CD patients do not achieve complete remission after 6 months of treatment with TNF-alpha blockers. Furthermore, 20% of CD patients treated with TNF-alpha blockers do not respond clinically to their primary biologic which is now referred to as primary non-response (PNR). Additionally, research demonstrates that an estimated 35% experience a loss of response (LOR) as biologics treatment progresses."[9]

   How come, for so many patients, these expensive biologic drugs either do not work from the beginning, or stop working eventually? The problem stems from immunogenicity.

3. **Immunogenicity Problem and Rejection Response.**

   What is immunogenicity?

   It's the ability of a foreign substance to provoke an immune response. Sometimes, an IBD patient has an abnormal immune response to biologic drugs. In this case, the patient's immune system forms antibodies that fight the medication.

You may wonder, how many biologics trigger this rejection response in IBD patients? The answer is shocking - *all of them do.*

According to a lead researcher Dr. Séverine Vermeire from the Department of Gastroenterology in University Hospitals Leuven in Belgium: "Immunogenicity occurs with all six of the biologic agents in patients with IBD".[10]

4. **IBD patients stop responding to biologics over time.**

Dr. Russell D. Cohen, director of the Inflammatory Bowel Disease Center at The University of Chicago Medicine states:

"Loss of response to biologic agents is a common situation faced by gastroenterologists".

He talks about this problem in his paper "What to Do When Biologic Agents Are Not Working in IBD patients."[11]

Lead researcher S. Kansal from Murdoch Children's Research Institute in Melbourne, Australia states in his scientific review:

"Biologic agents are limited by loss of efficacy over time due to the development of antibodies, as well as a risk of local reactions, anaphylaxis, and vasculitis. Moreover the reported risk of lymphomas especially in young adult males on concomitant Azathioprine and infliximab, albeit low, further limits their use."[6]

Side Effects

Fungal infections

Before you take another TNF inhibitor medication, you absolutely must know that these medications can increase your risk for infections, specifically fungal infections.[5]

TNF inhibitors include the following:

- Adalimumab (Humira®)
- Certolizumab pegol (Cimzia®)
- Etanercept (Enbrel®)
- Golimumab (Simponi®)
- Infliximab (Remicade®)

Here is the CDC's list of serious fungal infections:

- Histoplasmosis
- Cryptococcosis
- Coccidioidomycosis
- Invasive Candida infection
- Pneumocystis pneumonia
- Invasive aspergillosis

Also, biologics can cause serious health problems such as tuberculosis, pneumonia, herpes, multiple sclerosis, Parkinson's disease, increased incidence of skin cancer and malignant lymphoma, congestive heart failure, and liver disease.[12]

What happens if biologics fail

When treatment with biologics fails to control IBD flares, doctors recommend surgery. Surgery is also recommended when a patient stops responding to all drugs, and the disease gets out of control.

#5 Antibiotics

What are they & how do they work?

Antibiotics are medications that fight bacterial infections. Antibiotics are used to kill bacteria and/or inhibit bacterial growth.

Antibiotics are the drug of choice when treating intestinal inflammation and infections in IBD. For example, in Crohn's disease, antibiotics may be used in patients who have abscesses (pockets of pus), or fistulae (abnormal connection of the diseased bowel to another body part like the skin, bladder, vagina, or another piece of bowel), as these complications are impacted by bacteria.

Finally, ulcerative colitis patients who have a "J-pouch" after colectomy, can develop pouchitis (inflammation in the pouch). Pouchitis is often effectively managed with antibiotics.

Also, antibiotics are often used for eliminating parasitic infections.

Examples

Here are 5 antibiotics that are often prescribed in IBD:

- Rifaximin (Xifaxan®)
- Ampicillin (Omnipen®)
- Ciprofloxacin (Cipro®)
- Metronidazole (Flagyl®)
- Vancomycin (Vancomycin®)

Drawbacks

While antibiotics do treat infections, taking antibiotics may make you more susceptible to new bacterial infections. In the intestines, there live trillions of microorganisms (microbiota) that work together to maintain optimum health in the body.

C. difficile Infection Following Antibiotics Use

Long and/or frequent use of antibiotics disrupts the healthy equilibrium of intestinal microbiota, leading to destruction of good bacteria that allows pathogenic bacteria, like C. difficile, to take over.

What is the treatment for C. difficile?

You guessed it - another round of antibiotics.

It's a vicious circle of antibiotic treatment.

Patients with IBD are especially vulnerable to C. difficile infections. Study results from the Inflammatory Bowel Disease Center in Medical College of Wisconsin "have shown that over half of C. difficile-infected IBD patients will require hospitalization and the colectomy rate may approach 20%."[13, 14]

Side effects

Antibiotics are associated with numerous side effects: nausea, vomiting, loss of appetite, rash, diarrhea, dizziness, and headaches - even in healthy people. Imagine what can happen to IBD patients with impaired gut functions if they take antibiotics long-term.

The most serious problem encountered with antibiotic use is the potential to develop antibiotic resistance. This means that the bacteria mutate in a way that either reduces or defeats the effectiveness of the antibiotics. If this happens, harmful bacteria can multiply uncontrollably, causing more harm to the patient.

Antibiotic resistance in IBD was demonstrated in 2 studies.

Study 1: The antibiotic Ciprofloxacin was used in the treatment of intra-abdominal abscesses of patients with Crohn's disease (CD). This study analyzed 78 CD patients with intra-abdominal abscesses, who had their abscesses drained and analyzed. Conclusions of the study: "When gram-negative aerobes were isolated from abscesses in CD patients, more than two thirds were resistant to ciprofloxacin. Providers should consider this high rate of ciprofloxacin resistance when choosing first-line antibiotic treatment for CD-related intra-abdominal abscesses."[15]

Study 2: The antibiotic Rifaximin was used in the treatment of E. coli, a bacteria known to trigger the IBD process. E. coli strains were isolated from the lining of the small intestine (ileum) of 48 patients with IBD. Resistance to rifaximin was present in 12 out of 48 patients. Conclusion of the study: "Resistance correlated with prior rifaximin treatment."[16]

So, what happens if drugs don't work to solve your IBD? Conventional medicine offers only one other solution: surgery.

Treatment #2: Surgery

Years ago, when drugs stopped working on me, my own colitis was labeled "unmanageable". As a last resort, my doctors proposed surgery. Their idea of a cure was colectomy - removal of my colon.

With surgery, the diseased parts of the small and/or large intestine are cut out. Since ulcerative colitis is limited to the colon, GI doctors practicing conventional medicine will tell you that colectomy (surgery that removes the entire colon) is the only cure for the disease. This was the case when I was offered a colectomy more than 30 years ago.

Amazingly, today, decades later, conventional medicine remains the same. It's their simple formula for an IBD cure:

NO COLON = NO PROBLEM.

When is surgery necessary?

In some instances, colon surgery may be necessary to save a patient's life. Here are cases where surgery is essential:

1. **Toxic megacolon:** When the colon expands and the bowels cannot be emptied, this results in gas and feces buildup in the colon. This can trigger a colon rupture. If that happens, bacteria-laden stool would move freely into the abdomen, possibly causing sepsis, organ failure, and death.
2. **Bowel obstruction:** When the colon is blocked by cancerous tumors or narrowing of the intestine, the obstruction does not allow stool, gas, and fluids to move normally inside the colon. This cuts off the blood supply to the intestinal tissues. Symptoms of bowel obstruction include severe abdominal pain, cramps, bloating, vomiting, diarrhea, or constipation.
3. **Perforation of the colon:** When an inflamed colon has a deep ulcer, it can create a hole in the intestinal wall. Stool can leak into the abdomen, potentially causing sepsis, organ failure, and death.
4. **Dysplasia:** When abnormal cells develop in the lining of the colon and rectum, this is called dysplasia, and colorectal cancer may develop.
5. **Colon cancer:** When a cancerous tumor is present, it must be removed surgically.
6. **Thickening of the Intestinal Wall:** When the intestinal wall thickens, it narrows the intestinal passageway, which in time can result in intestinal obstruction preventing the normal flow of stool.

These are examples of conditions where surgery is necessary. However, is surgery the ultimate solution to all cases of Crohn's and colitis?

Many people suffering for years with IBD start to consider surgical removal of their diseased intestines. They hope surgery will be the final "cure". They hope that after they get rid of their colon, all their digestive problems will be gone. Poof, just disappear...

I, and many of my clients, have faced this same dilemma at some point in our lives. And so, I MUST SHARE with you a few facts to consider before making this life-changing decision.

Side effects

It turns out, there are many possible side effects and complications that can result from surgery.

Dr. Ochsenkühn (IBD center of the University of Munich) and Dr. D'Haens (Academic Medical Centre, Amsterdam) say:

> *"Although it is often stated that by removing the colon normal life can be restored in all patients, this is unfortunately rarely the case. A variety of complications can occur after surgery. Pouchitis, pouch leakage, pelvic abscesses, pouch fistulae, small bowel obstruction, anastomotic stricture, postoperative bleeding, fecal incontinence, sexual dysfunction and female infertility are frequent."*[17]

Let's look at some of the side effects of surgery:

Side Effect #1: After surgery, you can have postoperative bleeding. This is internal bleeding and would require more surgery.

Side Effect #2: After surgery, you can suffer from fecal incontinence. The colon helps to form feces. So, if your colon is removed, you might have diarrhea multiple times a day, including at night. A Swiss study of 107 UC patients evaluated after colon surgery found that "66% of patients reported 5-10 bowel movements per day and 73% had at least one movement during the night."[17]

That's a lot of running to the bathroom, which can result in electrolyte & vitamin deficiency, chronic fatigue, and weight loss. Without a colon, you give up essential functions such as processing fiber, and absorption of water, electrolytes, vitamins, and other nutrients.

Side Effect #3: After surgery, you may have intestinal obstruction. This can happen anytime within a few months or a few years after the surgery, as a result of scarring of the intestinal tissue. It's a very painful condition and requires more surgery.

Side Effect #4: After surgery, you can suffer from the most serious complication - leakage of bowel contents into your abdomen, from the two portions of your intestines that have been sewn together. This can result in abdominal pain, infection, and peritonitis, requiring more surgery and powerful antibiotic therapy.

Side Effect #5: After surgery, you might suffer from pouchitis, inflammation of the ileal pouch. Symptoms include diarrhea, abdominal cramps, and rectal bleeding.

According to Dr. Ofer Ben-Bassat from the IBD Center in Mount Sinai Hospital in Toronto:

> *"Up to 50% of patients can be expected to experience at least one episode of pouchitis, and most of these patients will experience at least one additional acute episode within 2 years."*[18]

Side Effect #6: After some types of colon surgery, the doctors set you up for a colostomy bag. This involves having a hole in your abdominal wall, connected to a bag for collecting your feces. Many patients have problems with feces leaking out of their colostomy bag.

Side Effect #7: After colectomy, you may also have sexual complications. If you are a woman, you can experience pain during intercourse due to scar tissue. If you are a man, you may stop having normal erections or normal ejaculation.

Side Effect #8: After ileostomy, you might experience recurrent prolapsed ileostomy. In an ileostomy, the large intestine is surgically cut out. Then, the ileum (the end of the small intestine) is rerouted to the surface of the abdomen, where a hole is constructed during surgery.

The tip of the ileum sticks out of the hole and is used to move feces out of the body, which goes into a special ileostomy bag. The most common complication of ileostomy is prolapse. It's when the tip of the ileum protrudes out of the hole in the abdomen. It looks scary because it appears like the intestine is literally hanging out. Additional surgery is required if the prolapse is too large.

Ileostomy prolapse is a recurrent problem and "occurs in 22% of adults and 38% of children" according to Professor K. Bielecki from the Department of General and Gastroenterological Surgery, Orlowski Hospital, Warsaw, Poland.[19]

I've linked a video about prolapsed ileostomy care, to give an idea of what you might be dealing with. Watch here:
http://knowyourgut.com/resources/

Side effect #9: Multiple bowel surgeries mean that a large portion of the intestine is removed. This leads to another severe problem called Short Bowel Syndrome. This syndrome describes a great reduction in a patient's ability to absorb carbohydrates, fats, vitamins, minerals, and fluids. This results in severe diarrhea, dehydration, malnutrition, malabsorption, and undesired weight loss.

As you can see, surgery comes with the potential for a lot of problems. And what happens if surgery fails? That's it - you either get another surgery, or you die.

Are drugs and surgery the only solutions to IBD?

Dr. David J. Maron (Department of Colorectal Surgery Cleveland Clinic in Florida) and Dr. Robert Lewis (Department of Surgery in University of Pennsylvania in Philadelphia) discuss "Efficacy and Complications of Surgery for Crohn's Disease". Here what they say:

> *"between 70% and 90% of patients with Crohn's disease will require surgery during their lifetime". "Indications for surgery include complications from strictures, intra-abdominal and perianal fistulas, intestinal perforation, intra-abdominal abscess, gastrointestinal bleeding, malignancy, and growth restriction in children."*[20]

I hope by now, you understand that there is no magic pill that can cure IBD. That is why it's so important to address the root causes of your disease.

If drugs aren't working for you, consider another option – Flare Stopper System. It can help you stop your IBD flare.

Realize this - if you don't change your diet & lifestyle, and if you don't address the root cause of your disease, the inflammation will continue. The disease will progress.

You will be likely forced to undergo painful, repetitive surgeries. If a doctor removes your colon, it's difficult to get back to restoration of your health and a normal life. You might be burdened with problems forever.

So, think twice before you decide to remove your colon. If you are looking to regain full control of your life, and truly heal your digestive system, surgery may not be the answer.

Don't get me wrong. I am NOT rejecting colectomy, or any other necessary surgery for intestinal obstructions or perforation, perianal and intra-abdominal fistulas and colon malignancy. In some cases, surgery is necessary and the only choice to save a patient's life. But the word "necessary" is key here.

You may feel that your normal, healthy life has been stolen from you by IBD. And you may think that drugs & surgery are your only salvation. However, your choice must ultimately be made only after considering ALL facts and possibilities. Search beyond conventional answers, seek second and third opinions, and consider EVERY possible solution before making an irreversible decision.

Please understand - removal of your colon does not stop the disease process, and most definitely does not restore your health. The truth is, after colectomy, your life will never be the same.

Some doctors say that removing the colon is a cure. According to the Merriam-Webster dictionary, the word "cure" means "something (such as a drug or medical treatment) that stops a disease and makes someone healthy again." I fully subscribe to this definition - a cure is not only elimination of symptoms, but a complete return to optimal health.

I do not believe that surgery is the cure for IBD patients whose condition is not life-threatening. Once you remove your vital organs, you cannot get them back. They are gone from your body FOREVER. The risk of multiple painful side effects stays with you FOREVER.

Remember: this is YOUR body, YOUR life, and YOUR decision. There are alternatives your doctor simply may not know about. You must learn why you got sick with IBD, understand the causes of the disease, and deal with the causes first. Remember, surgery only deals with effects.

I feel your pain. I've been there myself. I've suffered like you do now. I have seen this story repeat over and over again. So, I dedicated my life to developing the Flare Stopper System. Dealing with the root cause of IBD is what this book is about. You will learn concrete actions you can take to help your body heal itself.

References

[1] Chang-Tai Xu et al. "Drug Therapy for Ulcerative Colitis." *World J Gastroenterology*. 2004 Aug 15; 10(16): 2311–2317. Published online 2004 Aug 15. doi: 10.3748/wjg.v10.i16.2311 https://www.ncbi.nlm.nih.gov/pmc/articles/PMC4576279/

[2] Rogers, S.A. MD. (2000); pg147. No More Heartburn. Kensington

[3] https://www.accessdata.fda.gov/drugsatfda_docs/label/2009/007073s124lbl.pdf

[4] Matsuoka, Katsuyoshi et al. "Evidence-based clinical practice guidelines for inflammatory bowel disease." *Journal of gastroenterology* vol. 53,3 (2018): 305-353. doi:10.1007/s00535-018-1439-1
https://www.ncbi.nlm.nih.gov/pmc/articles/PMC5847182/

[5] https://www.cdc.gov/fungal/infections/immune-system.html

[6] S. Kansal et al. "Enteral Nutrition in Crohn's Disease: An Underused Therapy." *Gastroenterol Res Pract*. 2013; 2013: 482108. Published online 2013 Dec 5. doi: 10.1155/2013/482108
https://www.ncbi.nlm.nih.gov/pmc/articles/PMC3870077/

[7] https://pharmaceutical-journal.com/article/research/management-of-patients-with-inflammatory-bowel-disease-current-and-future-treatments

[8] Helen Yu et al. "Market Share and Costs of Biologic Therapies for Inflammatory Bowel Disease in the United States" *Aliment Pharmacol Ther*. 2018 Feb; 47(3): 364–370. Published online 2017 Nov 22. doi: 10.1111/apt.14430.

[9] https://www.alpco.com/challenges-when-treating-ibd-with-biologics

[10] Vermeire, Séverine et al. "Immunogenicity of biologics in inflammatory bowel disease." *Therapeutic advances in gastroenterology* vol. 11 1756283X17750355. 21 Jan. 2018, doi:10.1177/1756283X17750355

[11] Sushila R. Dalal, MD, and Russell D. Cohen, MD. "What to Do When Biologic Agents Are Not Working in Inflammatory Bowel Disease Patients". Gastroenterol Hepatol (N Y). 2015 Oct; 11(10): 657–665.

[12] Park SC, Jeen YT. "Anti-integrin therapy for inflammatory bowel disease." *World J Gastroenterol* 2018; 24(17): 1868-1880
www.ncbi.nlm.nih.gov/pmc/articles/PMC5937204/

[13] Issa M, Ananthakrishnan AN, Binion DG. "Clostridium difficile and inflammatory bowel disease." *Inflamm Bowel Dis*. 2008 Oct;14(10):1432-42. doi: 10.1002/ibd.20500. PMID: 18484669.

[14] Adam M. Berg, MD, Ciarán P. Kelly, MD, Francis A. Farraye, MD, MSc, "Clostridium difficile Infection in the Inflammatory Bowel Disease Patient". *Inflammatory Bowel Diseases*, Volume 19, Issue 1, 1 January 2013, Pages 194–204,
https://doi.org/10.1002/ibd.22964

[15] Park SK, Kim KJ, Lee SO, Yang DH, Jung KW, Duk Ye B, Byeon JS, Myung SJ, Yang SK, Kim JH, Sik Yu C. "Ciprofloxacin usage and bacterial resistance patterns in Crohn's disease patients with abscesses." *J Clin Gastroenterol*. 2014 Sep;48(8):703-7. doi: 10.1097/MCG.0000000000000024. PMID: 24296421.

[16] Kothary V, Scherl EJ, Bosworth B, et al. "Rifaximin resistance in Escherichia coli associated with inflammatory bowel disease correlates with prior rifaximin use, mutations in rpoB,

and activity of Phe-Arg-β-naphthylamide-inhibitable efflux pumps." *Antimicrobial Agents and Chemotherapy*. 2013 Feb;57(2):811-817. DOI: 10.1128/aac.02163-12.)

[17] Thomas Ochsenkühn, Geert D'Haens. "Current misunderstandings in the management of ulcerative colitis." *Gut* 2011, 60:1294e1299. doi:10.1136/gut.2010.218180

[18] Steinhart, A Hillary, and Ofer Ben-Bassat. "Pouchitis: a practical guide." *Frontline gastroenterology* vol. 4,3 (2013): 198-204. doi:10.1136/flgastro-2012-100171

[19] Bielecki, K. "Recurrent ileostomy prolapse: is it a solved problem?" *Techniques in coloproctology* vol. 14,3 (2010): 283-4. doi:10.1007/s10151-010-0598-8

[20] Lewis, Robert T, and David J Maron. "Efficacy and complications of surgery for Crohn's disease." *Gastroenterology & hepatology* vol. 6,9 (2010): 587-96.

CHAPTER 7

The Flare Stopper™ System Program Overview

ARE YOU SICK AND TIRED OF SUFFERING FROM CROHN'S DISEASE AND ULCERATIVE COLITIS?

ARE CURRENT TREATMENTS NOT WORKING FOR YOU?

Then, my program is what you need to eliminate pain, stop bloody diarrhea, and take back control of the life you deserve! Keep in mind: if you stick to the program as instructed, you will achieve great results.

What are the goals of this program?

- Stop intestinal bleeding and diarrhea
- Support the body's healthy immune response
- Lower GI inflammation, promote rapid healing of intestinal ulcers and induce remission

What are the components of the program?

You'll find a chapter dedicated to each component of this program, including:

- The Flare Stopper™ Diet
- Supplements
- Therapies
  - Medicinal Clay™ Poultice
  - Ileocecal valve adjustment
  - Cleansing Enema and Retention Enemas
  - Rectal Ozone Insufflation

Each component of the program will be described in detail later in the book.

What should you expect during the program?

A combination of a special liquid, enteral diet (the Flare Stopper™ diet), anti-inflammatory herbal remedies, detoxing supplements can help you to heal and seal the inflamed and ulcerated gut lining.

You will also be doing gut-restoring therapies that will reduce colon toxicity, reset intestinal microbiome and jump start the process of gut healing.

So, please take time off work and school for the duration of the program. There will be some initial weight loss - do not be alarmed. After inflammation subsides and a new gut lining has grown, your overall digestion and food assimilation will be greatly improved. You will start gaining healthy weight fast.

What should you expect after completing the program?

The good news is that after you complete this system, your intestinal bleeding, diarrhea, abdominal pain, and cramps should stop. Expect to pass well-formed stools 1-3 times a day. The Flare Stopper™ Diet and anti-inflammatory and detoxification remedies and therapies work synergistically to eliminate chronic intestinal inflammation and restore normal immune function.

Program Testimonials

Check out these testimonials to hear about the experiences of IBD patients like you:

Charon - Ulcerative Colitis for 8 years

> *"Prior to the program I had up to 5 bowel movements a day, semi-formed, or diarrhea with blood. After following the program for 12 days, I reported to Galina: My stool is free and clear of blood. I am pooping just 1-2 times a day. No pain! No bloating! And no urges at night to run to the bathroom. It feels like a miracle."*

Penteteuch - Crohn's disease for 7 years

> *"My Crohn's symptoms stopped after being on your program for 14 days. This is after 7 years of being sick with flare ups even when I was taking medication. I had lots of gas, bleeding with diarrhea and mucus for up to 12 bowel movements a day. At one point, I was only 90 pounds. I had tried everything. I could not work, was in a hospital two times and was offered surgery. I said 'no'. Instead, I began following Galina's instructions. While the liquid meals are kind of restrictive, it is amazing how quickly my symptoms cleared: no pain, no cramping, no diarrhea, no blood in the stool. Galina's system really worked for me."*

How long will the program take?

The timing for recovery varies. Some patients experience full relief of their symptoms in as little as 7 days. Some need 14 days, and others require up to 30 days of being on the program to stop their flare. So, rather than counting days on the program, strive for results (meaning total resolution of symptoms).

Due to the severity of my own pancolitis, I had to stay on the program for 30 days to stop my flare. It was hard - but I did it. After completing the program, my life changed dramatically. I stopped running to the bathroom more than 15 times a day with bloody diarrhea and tons of mucus. I stopped having excruciating pain and spasms while going to the bathroom. Finally, I was free from my sad life of being in the bathroom most of the day. At last, I was passing solid, formed stool 1-2 times a day, free of blood and mucus. I regained my life and my freedom.

Challenges you may experience during the program

1. Increased discharge of mucus

As a result of intestinal cleansing and detoxification, mucoid plaque will be broken down and purged from your body. In IBD, the inflamed, spastic bowel can retain pounds of mucoid plaque which is a perfect breeding ground for pathogens. This plaque is thickened mucus with a gel-like consistency. When you start deep cleaning your intestines, you begin to remove mucoid plaque. So, it's normal to see increased mucus discharge with each stool. You can even observe your stool being fully wrapped in mucus. Some patients can discharge up to a cup of mucus a day. You should welcome this mucus flow because this will unclog your intestines and will improve your digestion and absorption in the long-term, thereby allowing your gut to heal.

2. Feeling weak, hungry, fatigued with muscle aches

It's normal to feel weak and or hungry during this phase because your body is undergoing major cleansing and detoxification. It is common for most people to experience muscle aches, headaches, and fatigue. Those are the symptoms that tell you your body is using its innate energy to cleanse, detox, and build new healthy tissues. You are initiating a true healing process; therefore, it is essential to give your body plenty of bed rest and lots of sleep to ensure fast recovery.

3. Weight Loss

Don't be alarmed with initial weight loss during this program. Once you heal your gut lining, your digestion and absorption will normalize, and you will rapidly gain weight.

The Good News

1. Bowel Movement Frequency

You can expect your bowel movement frequency to decrease significantly. Some of my patients had 10-15 bowel movements a day prior to starting the program. After the completion of the program, these patients enjoyed 2-3 healthy bowel movements a day, pain-free.

2. Bowel Movement Quality

You can expect your bowel movement quality to improve dramatically. Your bowel movements will transition from diarrhea with blood and chunks of mucus, to blood-free and mucus-free fully formed stool.

Here is a common misconception: most people assume that while being on a liquid diet, their stool should be liquid. This is NOT true if you are consuming soluble fiber. A liquid diet leaves minimal residue in your digestive tract, but soluble fiber can help form stool. In this program, you will be consuming soluble fiber in the form of psyllium husk and butternut squash soup. So, with the improvement of your intestinal flora, your stool will gradually become fully formed, bulky, and easy to pass.

Plus, your stool should be free of a pungent stench. If your stool stinks, it means that your gut still harbors toxins. Healthy poop doesn't smell. Expect to poop like a champion by the end of the program.

3. More Energy and Improved Immune Function

After completing the program, expect to have more energy and improved immune function because your colon is free from obstruction created by mucoid plaque, hardened feces, toxins, and pathogens.

The Flare Stopper Diet Fundamentals

The Flare Stopper Diet is a diet I created with tasty, gut-healing recipes that anyone can make at home with just a few basic ingredients.

During a flare, you do not want to overwhelm your digestive system with extra work. At the same time, your body needs nutrients to restore and rebuild itself.

This diet ensures that all the necessary electrolytes, amino acids, fats, vitamins, and minerals are delivered to your gut in the most absorbable form possible (fresh vegetable juices, herbal teas, alkaline water, gelatin, and soup).

The first 21 days you will consume only approved foods/drinks, and NOTHING ELSE. The duration of the diet can vary from 7 days to 30 days, or longer, depending on the age and condition of the patient. For simplicity, in this book I describe a 21-day plan - the average time required to get out of a flare.

How long should you stay on the diet?

You can stop doing The Flare Stopper Diet and move to a transitional diet when you see the following improvements:

- Stool is well-formed
- No intestinal bleeding
- No visible mucus in your stool
- No abdominal pain, spasms or diarrhea
- Stool frequency of no more than 2-3 bowel movements a day

Things to Remember:

1. **Discontinue Solid Foods**: to stop GI inflammation, use of solid foods MUST BE DISCONTINUED for the duration of the program.
2. **Plan to Rest:** plenty of bed rest will allow your body to build a new, healthy colon lining in the shortest possible time. Take time off your job and school to allow your body to rest and heal. You should not do this program while working or going to school. Make sure that during the program you get plenty of bed rest and luxurious, afternoon naps.
3. **Stop all Supplements:** discontinue taking all vitamins, minerals, and probiotics, except those recommended in the program. Binders, fillers, additives, and GMO ingredients that are often present in supplements can aggravate an already inflamed gut. When your gut is inflamed and bleeding, its capacity to digest and absorb nutrients is greatly reduced. Therefore, during this program, when your gut is healing, do NOT take any vitamins/minerals (especially in a hard pill form), B-complex vitamins, vitamin C, adaptogen herbs, digestive enzymes, or probiotics. Do not worry, you will get plenty of vitamins and minerals from freshly squeezed juices and soups.
4. **After the liquid diet, do not immediately move to solid foods:** do not start eating solid foods right after stopping the liquid diet. You must go through a transitional diet first (see section Transitional Diet). Attention: if this rule is ignored, the benefits of your liquid diet will be erased or possibly, your condition could worsen. Specifically, you could get very sick for days with stomach pain, bloating, nausea, constipation, or diarrhea. That's why I created the Transitional Diet - it's a safe bridge back to eating solid foods.

Foods You Can Eat and Drink

Consume ONLY allowed foods and drinks in The Flare Stopper Diet. Do not eat or drink anything that is not part of the program.

Important Note: All water must be boiled, including water for washing and disinfecting vegetables for juice. You must boil all water, even if it's bottled water.

How to Prepare for the Program

I know this seems complex and expensive. But this disease is complex, and the cost is astronomical in terms of money, time, and health. Investing effort now will pay off greatly in the future.

Supplies

Below is a list of supplies that you need to start the program. I've linked specific products on my website:
http://knowyourgut.com/resources/

Buy Enema Supplies

- 42 disposable fleet enemas
- Safe lubricants for enema nozzle:
    - Sterile lubricating jelly, or
    - Preparation H ointment

Buy Kitchen Supplies

- Juicer
- Slow cooker
- Blender
- Set of knives, 3 cutting boards, and a vegetable peeler
- French press (to brew black tea and green teas) and a strainer

- Glass lined thermos to brew Intestinal Comfort Tea™
- Non-toxic, ceramic pots and pans. Traditional nonstick cookware can be hazardous to your health because it is made with chemicals like PFAS and PFOA that can leach into your food during cooking.
- 6 bottles of 3% hydrogen peroxide (16 oz. each bottle)

Buy Food Supplies

Buy foods included in The Flare Stopper Diet:

- Carrots, celery, beets, lemons, fresh turmeric, turmeric powder, kale, romaine lettuce, parsley, pumpkin or butternut squash, garlic, onions, whole brown flaxseed, organic chicken, loose organic black tea, coconut oil, extra virgin olive oil, unsulfured blackstrap molasses, cayenne pepper, black pepper, Himalayan salt, baking soda (aluminum free). The above foods should be organic.

Buy Supplements
The Flare Stopper™ Kit:

- Colon Formula™
- Intestinal Comfort Tea™
- Medicinal Clay™
- Immunity G7 Formula™
- Cod Liver Oil
- Activated Charcoal
- Colon Cleansing Drink (psyllium husk + bentonite)
- Hydrolyzed Collagen or Gelatin
- Potassium Chloride
- Chlorophyll

In the next two chapters, you will see an example of the schedule you will follow for the next 21 days.

You will find details on the diet, supplements, and therapies in the next few chapters.

Schedule Overview

There are two phases in The Flare Stopper System:

Phase	Length	Purpose
Intro Phase	14 days	To Stop Bleeding, Diarrhea and Abdominal Pain
Transitional Phase	7 days	To Help Your Body to Build a Healthy Colon Lining

We'll go into details in the next few chapters on each phase's schedule, and the associated recipes, supplements, and therapies.

CHAPTER 8

Intro Phase Schedule (Days 1-14)

THE MAIN PURPOSE OF THIS PHASE IS TO STOP BLEEDING, DIARRHEA, and abdominal pain, lower overall inflammation, and induce remission.

This phase will last 14 days.

Note: when I was sick, I asked my family and friends to help me with my food prep and kitchen cleaning since I was too weak to do it myself. If you have family and friends, ask them for help. If you allow them to help you, they will feel that they are part of your life and your recovery. They will be happy to do it for you!

Prep Summary

Here is a summary of things you will prepare during this phase. You will also see these items listed in the Schedule table below.

Prep Daily, Morning

- Intestinal Comfort Tea (5 min prep + thermos brewing for 30 minutes to 4 hours)

- Organic flaxseed tea or CloroFlax Tea (prep 30 minutes, drink 3 cups daily)
- Colon Cleansing Drink (5 min prep)
- Electrolyte Drink (5 min prep)
- Vegetable Juice (30 min prep to disinfect vegetables & make juice)
- Cleansing Enema Solution (5 min prep)
- Retention Enema Solution (5 min prep + 1 hour brewing time)

Prep Daily, Evening

- Boil water (about 3 gallons) for disinfecting vegetables, for electrolyte drink, for intestinal cleansing drink, and for drinking (15 min prep)
- Peel vegetables for juicing & refrigerate for the morning (20 min prep)
- Peel butternut squash, about 2 pounds, remove seeds, slice & refrigerate for the morning (20 min prep)
- Prepare Medicinal Clay™ Drink (5 min prep)

Prep every 2 days

- Pumpkin/Butternut Squash Soup (20 min prep)
- Chicken Soup (20 min prep + cooking 2 hours)

Schedule

Time	Activity	Amount
6:55am	Drink warm alkaline water mixed with 1 Tablespoon of freshly squeezed lemon juice.	1 cup
7:00am	Prepare Galina's Electrolyte drink.	4 cups
7:05am	Prepare Intestinal Comfort™ tea.	3 cups
7:10am	Prepare Colon Cleansing drink.	1 cup

7:15am	Drink Galina's Electrolyte drink with 2 caps of Activated Charcoal	1 cup
8:00am	Drink Intestinal Comfort tea +Colon Cleansing drink	1 cup of each
8:10am	Prepare enema solution (for both: cleansing and retention enemas).	2 enemas
8:30am	Drink Medicinal Clay™ drink.	1 cup
8:45am	Prepare vegetable juice.	3-4 cups
9:15am	Drink vegetable juice with 1 teaspoon of cod liver oil. Take 2 capsules of Colon Formula	1 cup
9:30am	Prepare black tea with collagen or gelatin.	1 cup
9:45am	Drink black tea with collagen or gelatin.	1 cup
10:00am	Prepare flaxseed tea.	3 cups
10:30am	Drink flaxseed tea + Galina's Electrolyte Drink.	1 cup of each
10:40am	Prepare pumpkin soup. Refrigerate leftover soup.	1-2 cups
11:10am	Eat pumpkin soup.	1-2 cups
11:30am	Drink Galina's Electrolyte drink with 2 caps of Activated Charcoal	1 cup
11:45am	Drink Intestinal Comfort tea.	1 cup
12:00pm	Drink Medicinal Clay drink.	1 cup
12:10pm	Do enemas (both cleansing and retention).	1 of each
12:40pm	Drink vegetable juice with 1 teaspoon of cod liver oil. Take 2 capsules of Colon Formula	1 cup
1:00pm	Drink flaxseed tea, & drink black tea with collagen or gelatin.	1 cup
1:15pm	Eat chicken soup.	1-2 cups
1:30pm	Take an afternoon nap.	1 hr 30 min
3:00pm	Drink vegetable juice with 1 teaspoon of cod liver oil.	1 cup
3:30pm	Drink black tea with collagen or gelatin.	1 cup
3:45pm	Eat pumpkin soup.	1 bowl

4:00pm	Go for a slow walk / do gentle yoga / stretch.	1 hour
5:00pm	Drink Galina's Electrolyte drink with 2 caps of Activated Charcoal	2 cups
5:00pm	Prepare chicken soup. Simmer for about 2 hours. After soup is cooled, refrigerate leftovers.	8 cups
5:30pm	Drink Intestinal Comfort tea.	1 cup
5:45pm	Drink vegetable juice with 1 teaspoon of cod liver oil. Take 2 capsules of Colon Formula	1 cup
6:00pm	Eat pumpkin soup.	1-2 bowls
6:15pm	Drink flaxseed tea.	1 cup
6:30pm	Apply Medicinal Clay poultice.	1 application
7:00pm	Eat chicken soup.	1-2 cups
7:15pm	Drink Intestinal Comfort tea.	1 cup
7:30pm	Drink Medicinal Clay drink.	1 cup
8:30pm	Remove Medicinal Clay poultice.	1 removal
8:40pm	Drink Galina's Electrolyte drink.	1 cup
8:45pm	Peel vegetables for tomorrow's juice and Peel and slice butternut squash for tomorrow's soup.	
9:00pm	Drink Colon Cleansing drink + Galina's Electrolyte drink.	1 cup of each
9:15pm	Boil 3 gallons of water to let cool overnight. Prepare Medicinal Clay drink for tomorrow.	
9:30pm	Relaxation, meditation, bedtime.	

CHAPTER 9

Transitional Phase Schedule (Days 15-21)

THE MAIN PURPOSE OF THIS PHASE IS TO TRANSITION FROM A LIQUID diet to a solid food diet. The return to a normal eating schedule must be done slowly. This phase will allow time for your gastrointestinal system to readjust to absorption of solid foods and healthy digestion. If you ignore the transitional phase, you can experience abdominal pain, cramps, nausea, vomiting, diarrhea, or constipation.

This phase will last 7 days.

Prep Summary

Here is a summary of things you will prepare during this phase. You will also see these items listed in the Schedule table below.

Prep Daily, Morning

- Golden milk (drink 1 cup daily)
- Electrolyte Drink (prep 5 min; drink 2-4 cups daily)

- Organic flaxseed tea or CloroFlax Tea (prep 30 minutes, drink 3 cups daily)
- Colon Cleansing Drink (5 min; drink 2 times daily)
- Intestinal Comfort Tea (5 min prep + thermos brewing for at least 30 minutes, up to few hours; drink 3 cups daily)
- Fresh, raw vegetable Juice (disinfect vegetables & juice: 30 min; drink undiluted, up to 4 cups daily)
- Hydrolyzed Collagen drink mixed with water (prep 5 min; drink 1 cup daily)
- Cleansing Enema Solution (5 min)
- Retention Enema Solution (5 min prep + brewing time 1 hour)

Prep Daily, Evening

- Boil water (about 3 gallons) for disinfecting vegetables, for electrolyte drink, for intestinal cleansing drink and just drinking (15 min)
- Peel vegetables for juicing & refrigerate for the morning (20 min)
- Peel butternut squash, about 2 pounds, remove seeds and slice & refrigerate for the morning (20 min)

Prep every 2 days

- Pumpkin/Butternut Squash Soup (20 min prep)
- Blood building soup (10 min prep + cooking 30 minutes; eat 1-2 bowls)
- Chicken soup blended with boiled carrots and parsley root (20 min prep + cooking 2 hours; eat 1-2 bowls)

Prep every 3 days

- Bone Broth (Prep 20 minutes + cooking 10-12 hours; drink 2 cups daily; drink 1-2 cups daily; freeze extra broth)

Schedule

Time	Activity	Amount
6:55am	Drink warm alkaline water mixed with 1 Tablespoon of fresh lemon juice.	1 cup
7:00am	Prepare Electrolyte drink.	4 cups
7:05am	Prepare Intestinal Comfort™ tea.	3 cups
7:10am	Prepare Colon Cleansing drink.	1 cup
7:15am	Drink Colon Cleansing drink + Galina's Electrolyte drink.	1 cup of each
8:00am	Drink Intestinal Comfort™ tea.	1 cup
8:10am	Prepare enema solution (for both: cleansing and retention enemas).	2 enemas
8:30am	Eat chicken soup.	1-2 bowls
8:45am	Prepare vegetable juice.	3-4 cups
9:15am	Drink vegetable juice with 1 tablespoon of cod liver oil. Refrigerate the rest of the juice in a glass jar.	1 cup
9:30am	Prepare golden milk.	1 cup
9:45am	Drink golden milk.	1 cup
10:00am	Prepare flaxseed tea.	3 cups
10:30am	Drink flaxseed tea + Galina's electrolyte drink.	1 cup of each
10:40am	Prepare pumpkin soup. Refrigerate leftover soup.	1-2 cups
11:10am	Eat pumpkin soup. Take 1 capsule of Immunity G7 Formula	1-2 cups
11:30am	Drink Galina's Electrolyte drink.	1 cup
11:45am	Drink Intestinal Comfort tea.	1 cup
11:50pm	Prepare blood building soup.	
12:00pm	Drink water with collagen or gelatin.	1 cup
12:10pm	Do enemas (both cleansing and retention).	1 of each
12:40pm	Eat blood building soup.	1-2 bowls
1:00pm	Drink flaxseed tea.	1 cup

1:15pm	Drink vegetable juice with 1 tablespoon of cod liver oil.	1 cup
1:30pm	Take an afternoon nap.	1 hr 30 min
3:00pm	Drink vegetable juice with 1 tablespoon of cod liver oil.	1 cup
3:30pm	Drink bone broth.	1 cup
3:45pm	Eat pumpkin soup. Take 1 capsule of Immunity G7 Formula	1 bowl
4:00pm	Go for a slow walk / do gentle yoga / stretch.	1 hour
5:00pm	Prepare chicken soup. Simmer for about 2 hours. After soup is cooled, refrigerate leftovers.	8 cups
5:30pm	Drink Intestinal Comfort tea.	1 cup
5:40pm	Peel vegetables for tomorrow's juice and Peel and slice butternut squash for tomorrow's soup.	
5:45pm	Drink Vegetable juice with 1 teaspoon of cod liver oil.	1 cup
6:00pm	Eat pumpkin soup.	1-2 bowls
6:15pm	Drink flaxseed tea.	
6:30pm	Apply Medicinal Clay poultice.	1 application
7:00pm	Eat chicken soup. Take 1 capsule of Immunity G7 Formula	1-2 cups
8:00pm	Drink Galina's Electrolyte drink.	1 cup
8:30pm	Remove Medicinal Clay poultice.	1 removal
8:45pm	Prep bone broth & cook overnight in a slow cooker.	
9:00pm	Drink Colon Cleansing drink + Galina's Electrolyte drink.	1 cup of each
9:15pm	Boil water for tomorrow.	
9:30pm	Relaxation, meditation, bedtime.	

CHAPTER 10

The Flare Stopper Diet™

If you are in an active flare, you must start The Flare Stopper Diet ASAP (as soon as possible) for elimination of diarrhea, abdominal pain, and bleeding. The Flare Stopper Diet is a therapeutic diet that can help you reverse the IBD disease process and achieve gut healing you are looking for.

How do I know it will? Because it worked for me and many of my clients.

What is The Flare Stopper Diet?

The Flare Stopper Diet is a special liquid, enteral diet I designed for IBD patients who cannot eat solid food because they either feel too sick to eat normal meals or are afraid to eat due to abdominal pain, cramps, and diarrhea. Liquid meals mean less risk of irritating intestines that are inflamed, and/or have bleeding ulcers.

The Flare Stopper Diet is designed to induce remission in IBD patients, and it's super safe. It completely excludes any foods and substances like common food allergens and harmful additives/ingredients that could damage your gut in any way.

But The Flare Stopper Diet does not stop there. It supercharges your body with live enzymes, bioavailable vitamins/minerals, and easy to digest proteins, fats, and carbohydrates, ensuring healing from the inside out.

As Hippocrates said more than 2,000 years ago:" Let food be thy medicine, and medicine be thy food."

The Flare Stopper Diet is a short-term enteral nutrition diet, which means mostly liquid foods are taken through the mouth.

Diet duration can vary from 7 to 30 days, or longer, depending on the age and the condition of the patient. Some patients experience full relief from IBD symptoms after only 7 days of being on The Flare Stopper Diet, some after 14 days, while others may require up to 30 days or longer of being on this diet to induce remission.

For the purpose of this book, I recommend doing at least 21 days of The Flare Stopper Diet™. I personally have done The Flare Stopper Diet™ for 30 days, because I have been sick with a severe case of ulcerative pancolitis for many years. That's why it took me a whole month to stop my severe GI inflammation and bleeding.

You may be thinking, "Wow, 30 days of drinking liquids. I don't know if I can do it. "But if you knew that 1 month of The Flare Stopper Diet will help you regain full control of your digestive system, would you do it?

After years of suffering and numerous useless treatments and diets, I realized that it's much easier to do The Flare Stopper Diet for a month, than to be sick and miserable for the rest of my life. I tried so many things to get rid of my colitis, including commercial liquid enteral formulas. But it turned out that my own Enteral Nutrition diet was far more effective in healing my gut than all the anti-inflammatories, antibiotics, and steroid drugs I was prescribed.

After completing 30 days of The Flare Stopper Diet, drinking herbs, taking supplements and doing therapies discussed in this book, I stopped having diarrhea, bleeding, and cramps. And I began enjoying pain-free, healthy bowel movements. In short, I became a real pooping champion!

Years later, my numerous clients had similar success with The Flare Stopper Diet.

I know for a fact that The Flare Stopper Diet is one of the most effective tools you can use to repair your gut wall lining, regulate your intestinal microflora, and take control of your seemingly uncontrollable disease!

Realize this: you must be patient with your body! It takes time for your body to heal and restore when using diet, anti-inflammatory herbs, and gut-healing therapies.

What is Commercial Enteral Nutrition?

In a hospital setting, Enteral Nutrition refers to a special liquid diet given to patients by mouth who cannot eat solid food. Most of these are commercial meal replacement drinks packaged in 8-ounce cans.

Doctors prescribe them to patients with ulcerative colitis and Crohn's disease who cannot tolerate solid food, or who have lost a lot of weight due to malnutrition and malabsorption.

While commercial Enteral Nutrition formulas can help some patients achieve remission, many of the clients I have seen refused to drink these formulas because of the taste and side effects. In fact, that's when I observed that some clients reacted to these commercial formulas the same way I did - with bloating and diarrhea.

Why did I create The Flare Stopper Diet™?

More than 30 years ago, I was forced to create my own version of an enteral diet or special liquid diet because commercial formulas simply did not work for me.

The commercial enteral formulas had a horrible taste (which I decided to endure for the sake of better health), and their ingredients created more problems for me.

After a thorough investigation of different commercial formulas, I realized that in addition to the tremendous amount of sugars and artificial sweeteners that threw off the balance in my sensitive gut, they contained a whole array of chemicals that later were scientifically proven as harmful for IBD.

As in the case of conventional IBD drugs, I found myself in the group of "unlucky" patients who are super sensitive to the synthetic compounds added to these formulas. So, you see, I created The Flare Stopper Diet not just because of professional curiosity; I did it out of desperate necessity.

I knew then that the idea of an enteral (liquid) diet made sense for the simple reason of letting your gut work easier during flares, allowing for the healing process to start.

Why The Flare Stopper Diet works?

Eating The Flare Stopper Diet means taking liquid meals with less risk of irritating intestines that are inflamed and bleeding. When you eat normal meals of solid foods, they go right through you without being properly absorbed. Nothing stays in.

Please, understand the following fact: a liquid diet is very different from starving yourself, which deprives you of nourishment and creates extreme deficiencies of nutrients. An enteral diet provides calories, protein, carbohydrates, fats, vitamins, and minerals in easy to digest form. It also accelerates the healing process of the intestinal lining and promotes natural recovery from IBD symptoms in a short period of time.

The following scientific studies show that Enteral Nutrition can be an effective treatment for IBD patients.

Scientific Studies Confirm Benefits of Enteral Nutrition for IBD

Since 1969, Enteral Nutrition formulas have been used as a treatment for patients with IBD. Here are the findings of world-renowned doctors and medical scientists.

1. Enteral nutrition can induce remission.

Dr. John Hunter from the UK reports that patients' ability to digest and absorb foods drastically improves while on Enteral Nutrition. He states:

> *"Overall, the results of enteral feedings are excellent with 80-100% of compliant patients going into full remission within 2-3 weeks. Such results compare favourably with those achieved by treatment of Crohn's disease with immunosuppression."*[1]

In Japan, Crohn's disease patients are treated first with Enteral Nutrition. This methodology is widely used by Japanese doctors since it has been proven repeatedly that Enteral Nutrition can induce remission and heal colon ulcers quickly.[2]

2. Enteral Nutrition can help maintain remission.

Ten studies were reviewed by doctors from the Inflammatory Bowel Disease Center at Yokkaichi Social Insurance Hospital in Japan. Their conclusion was that "Enteral nutrition (EN) may be useful for maintaining remission in patients with CD". They compared "outcomes between patients who received EN and those who did not. The clinical remission rate was significantly higher in those with EN in all seven studies."[3]

3. Enteral Nutrition improves bone density and lowers inflammation.

Researchers from Federal University in Bahia, Brazil identified that IBD patients, both adults and children, have increased risk of bone fractures due to bone loss (osteopenia and osteoporosis). This happens as a result of chronic inflammation, malnutrition, vitamin D deficiency, frequent and prolonged use of steroids, and post-surgery effects.

Furthermore, it was noted that "IBD patients with ostomy are at higher risk for bone loss, and these patients should be monitored closely, especially patients with risk factors, such as low BMI and a previous history of fractures."[4]

Enteral nutrition can be a solution for patients who experience serious bone loss and continuous inflammation.

A study on children with active Crohn's was conducted at the Stollery Children's Hospital in Edmonton, Alberta. Data was collected on the effects of Exclusive Enteral Nutrition (EEN) versus steroids in children with Crohn's disease (average age about 13 years).

In this study, 36 kids with Crohn's disease were given EEN, and 69 received corticosteroids. Remission rates were about 89% in the EEN group versus 91% in the steroid group. 34 patients were given a bone density scan test at the time of initial diagnosis, and again 12 months later. Change in bone mineral density was better for EEN patients than for patients on steroids.

The Bottom Line: enteral nutrition results in better bone mass density and "should be preferred to corticosteroids as first-line therapy for induction of remission in pediatric CD."[5]

4. Enteral nutrition can be used as an alternative to steroids.

According to Dr. Arun Swaminath, from the Gastroenterology division at Lenox Hill Hospital in NYC, Enteral Nutrition can be as effective as corticosteroids for inducing remission in children with Crohn's disease. Moreover, exclusive Enteral Nutrition may work better than steroids in healing the intestinal lining in Crohn's patients. Dr. Swaminath based her conclusion on 8 studies totaling 451 patients.[6]

For decades, doctors in Europe have proven repeatedly that Enteral Nutrition can be as effective as steroids in inducing remission in Crohn's disease and ulcerative colitis.

More than 30 years ago, the British Medical Journal published a study where Enteral Nutrition (aka elemental diet) was used as a primary treatment for patients with acute Crohn's disease.

In this study "21 acutely ill patients with Crohn's disease were randomized to receive either prednisolone or Enteral Nutrition (Vivonex elemental formula) for 4 weeks. Patients were evaluated at 4 and 12 weeks of the program."

The results of the study were amazing: Enteral Nutrition in the form of an elemental diet has been proven as a safe and effective treatment for acute Crohn's disease.

European doctors concluded that the elemental diet "offers a therapeutically effective non-toxic alternative to conventional surgery and drugs."[7]

Summary of Enteral Nutrition Benefits:

1. It can induce remission
2. It can help to maintain remission
3. It can be used as an alternative to steroids
4. It improves bone health and lowers inflammation
5. It is a safe and effective treatment for IBD; has practically no side effects

Why haven't you heard about Enteral Nutrition from your GI doctor?

Sadly, in the US very few GI doctors use Enteral Nutrition for IBD treatment. Here are the statistics on usage of nutrition therapy in the U.S. vs. Europe:

> *"While 62% of European gastroenterologists use nutrition therapy as the first line of treatment for the management of active Crohn's disease in children, only 4% of U.S. gastroenterologists use it. Most American gastroenterologists prefer to use drugs such as steroids and azathioprine instead of a diet."*[8]

A shocking difference in usage of nutrition therapy - 62% in Europe vs 4% in the U.S.!

That is why very few IBD patients in the U.S. know about the benefits of an Enteral Nutrition diet and how to use this simple, very effective diet to promote GI healing.

Also, GI doctors in the U.S. believe that compliance with the Enteral Nutrition diet is too low because patients feel restricted in their food choices and patients must drink the same formula for 4-6 weeks, which is pretty monotonous.

So, what can go wrong with Commercial Enteral Nutrition?

The above findings on Enteral Nutrition's benefits were very encouraging; they made sense to me. Nevertheless, my numerous attempts to stay on this diet using various commercial formulas always ended up worsening my condition. To add insult to injury, the commercial formulas tasted awful.

I knew something was missing from the Enteral Nutrition liquid diet. I loved the idea - but not the commercially available formulas. Because certain ingredients in these formulas worked against my gut healing, I again thought of myself as a super-sensitive freak.

Years later, I realized I was not a "super-sensitive freak". I was not alone; these reactions were not rare. Many other IBD sufferers experienced similar side effects that made their Enteral Nutrition diet ineffective. My research resulted in a list of possible ingredient offenders to be aware of:

1. **Glucose Syrup** (aka corn syrup in the U.S.) has as much nutritional value as table sugar. It can cause fermentation, bloating, and diarrhea in IBD patients with active Crohn's and Colitis.

2. **Sucrose** is another name for white table sugar. Sucrose is a combination of fructose and glucose. Both glucose syrup and sucrose are simple refined sugars, which can make the body's pH highly acidic. Furthermore, sugar feeds harmful bacteria and yeast like Candida in your gut. This, in turn, can cause more bloating, abdominal pain, and diarrhea. Furthermore, sugar used in these drinks is likely made from GMO beets. So, it's better to avoid products with refined sugar, especially during a flare.

3. **GMO-based ingredients** such as soy derivatives (soybean oil, soy protein isolate, soy lecithin), corn oil, corn starch,

maltodextrin, canola oil, dextrose, and citric acid are often added to commercial formulas. That presents a problem for IBD patients.

According to The Integrative Physician group in Scottsdale, Arizona: "Ultimately, GMOs create bowel hypersensitivity, increase inflammation and damage the intestinal lining. This makes IBD cases much worse, as they contribute to and in some cases, may actually trigger these diseases."[9]

4. **Artificial colors and flavors** are added to some EN formulas to improve their taste and color. According to the Center for Science for the Public Interest (CSPI), artificial colors (food dyes) should be banned because they are linked to cancer, allergies, and hyperactivity in children.[10]

5. **Carrageenan** is a thickener used in some EN formulas to add texture, increase viscosity, and keep ingredients from separating. It's a fact - carrageenan can cause inflammation and intestinal ulcers. Thirty years ago, scientists from the Department of Pathology in University of Liverpool, UK, conducted a study on carrageenan. In this study, young guinea pigs were given fluids containing carrageenan at a 1.2% and 3% concentration over a 2-week period. After just 4 days of drinking 3% carrageenan solution, 100% of the guinea pigs had developed ulcers in the colon, consistent with ulcerative colitis.[11]

   Imagine what carrageenan can do to your gut when you already have gut inflammation and bleeding ulcers.

Carrageenan can Actually Worsen Your Condition and Sabotage Your Recovery

Doctor J.K. Tobacman demonstrated in his 2012 study that consuming carrageenan has been associated with development of ulcerative colitis and malignant intestinal tumors in animals who ate carrageenan for less than 18 months.[12]

Despite these studies, you still can find carrageenan in elemental formulas prescribed for patients with ulcerative colitis and Crohn's disease.

You should know that carrageenan is widely used in many foods such as ice cream, candy bars, almond milk, chocolate milk, baby formula, whipped cream, cottage cheese, sour cream, yogurt, half-and-half, coffee creamers, soy-based coffee drinks, etc.

With all this in mind, check out the list of ingredients in four leading EN formulas. The problematic ingredients for IBD people during a flare are underlined.

1. **Vivonex RTF Elemental Formula Ingredients:** Water, Maltodextrin and less than 2% of Modified Cornstarch, L-Lysine Acetate, L-Leucine, Soybean Oil, L-Arginine, L-Glutamic Acid, Medium Chain Triglycerides (from Coconut and/or Palm Kernel Oil), Calcium Glycerophosphate, L-Threonine, L-Phenylalanine, L-Valine, L- Isoleucine, L-Proline, L-Histidine Hydrochloride, L-Methionine, Glycine, L-Tryptophan, Carrageenan, Dextrose, Potassium Citrate, Magnesium Sulfate, Sodium Citrate, L-Aspartic Acid, Citric Acid, L-Serine, Choline Bitartrate, L-Alanine, Sodium Hexametaphosphate, Ascorbic Acid, Salt, Potassium Chloride, L-Tyrosine, Taurine, L-Carnitine, L-Cystine, Alpha-Tocopheryl Acetate, Ferric Orthophosphate, Zinc Sulfate, Niacinamide, Vitamin A Palmitate, Calcium Pantothenate, Copper Gluconate, Manganese Sulfate, Pyridoxine Hydrochloride, Vitamin D3, Thiamine Hydrochloride, Riboflavin, Folic Acid, Chromium Chloride, Biotin, Potassium Iodide, Sodium Molybdate, Sodium Selenite, Phytonadione, Vitamin B12.
2. **Modulen IBD Ingredients:** Glucose syrup, Casein, Sucrose, Milk fat, Medium chain triglycerides, Corn oil, Emulsifier (Soya lecithin), Acidity regulator (Potassium hydroxide), Vitamins and Minerals.
3. **Peptamen Junior for Kids Ingredients:** Ingredients (Vanilla): Water, Maltodextrin, Enzymatically Hydrolyzed Whey Protein (From Milk), Sugar, Medium Chain Triglycerides (From Coconut And/Or Palm Kernel Oil) And Less Than 2% Of Cornstarch, Soybean Oil, Canola Oil, Calcium Phosphate, Soy Lecithin,

Guar Gum, Magnesium Chloride, Potassium Chloride, Sodium Phosphate, Potassium Citrate, Sodium Ascorbate, Natural And Artificial Flavor, Salt, Choline Chloride, Calcium Citrate, Potassium Phosphate, Acesulfame Potassium (Sweetener), Taurine, Alpha-Tocopheryl Acetate, Magnesium Oxide, Inositol, L-Carnitine, Ferrous Sulfate, Sucralose (Sweetener), Zinc Sulfate, Calcium Pantothenate, Niacinamide, Vitamin A Palmitate, Vitamin D3, Phytonadione, Thiamine Mononitrate, Manganese Sulfate, Pyridoxine Hydrochloride, Riboflavin, Copper Sulfate, Citric Acid, Beta-Carotene, Folic Acid, Biotin, Potassium Iodide, Chromium Chloride, Vitamin B12, Sodium Selenate. Contains: Milk And Soy Ingredients.

4. **Ensure Plus Strawberry Ready to Drink Ingredients:** Water, Corn Maltodextrin, Sugar, Milk Protein Concentrate, Canola Oil, Soy Protein Isolate, Corn Oil, Pea Protein Concentrate. Less than 0.5% of the Following: Magnesium Phosphate, Potassium Citrate, Natural & Artificial Flavor, Soy Lecithin, Sodium Citrate, Potassium Chloride, Calcium Phosphate, Calcium Carbonate, Salt, Choline Chloride, Ascorbic Acid, Potassium Hydroxide, Carrageenan, Ferrous Sulfate, dl-Alpha-Tocopheryl Acetate, Zinc Sulfate, Niacinamide, Manganese Sulfate, Calcium Pantothenate, FD&C Red #3, Cupric Sulfate, Vitamin A Palmitate, Thiamine Chloride Hydrochloride, Pyridoxine Hydrochloride, Riboflavin, Chromium Chloride, Folic Acid, Sodium Molybdate, Biotin, Sodium Selenate, Potassium Iodide, Phylloquinone, Vitamin D3, and Cyanocobalamin. Contains milk and soy ingredients.

Interesting, isn't it? No wonder some IBD people have issues with commercial enteral nutrition formulas.

The Flare Stopper Diet is the Way!

The ingredients present in commercial formulas worked against my healing. So, I was forced to look for a better alternative. That is how The Flare Stopper Diet was born.

Unlike commercial enteral formulas, The Flare Stopper Diet was designed to go beyond just providing calories and nutrients. It was designed with the mindset that we should use food as medicine. The Flare Stopper Diet provides the benefits of enteral, liquid nutrition WITHOUT the potentially harmful chemicals, sugar, and GMO ingredients found in commercial formulas.

The Flare Stopper Diet contains a wide array of plant-based phytonutrients, plus live enzymes, bioavailable vitamins, and minerals derived from whole, organic, fresh foods created by mother nature. This diet provides foods that are good for you. Many of my clients have seen great results after doing The Flare Stopper Diet for just 7 days.

The Flare Stopper Diet helped many of my IBD clients get out of severe, long-term flares after trying and failing numerous diets, natural supplements, and even powerful prescription drugs. Implemented together with other modalities in my program, this diet helps resolve intestinal inflammation in the shortest time possible, while assisting you in achieving quick remission naturally.

With The Flare Stopper Diet, you will not only stop running to the bathroom - you will also experience relief from stomach pain and abdominal spasms. Moreover, you'll push your body toward total revitalization of all your organs. This will result in fast recovery from your current flare. Getting well is easy when you start applying dietary principles that work.

What The Flare Stopper Diet Can Do for You:

- Allow your gut to rest and heal
- Help your body build a healthy, new colon lining
- Induce remission in some people with IBD in just 7 days
- Lower inflammation and enhance absorption of nutrients
- Promote GI healing in IBD people who do not respond to steroids
- Provide easy to digest nutrients, vitamins, minerals, and enzymes

- Enhance absorption of nutrients and reduce pain level in the body

3 Reasons Why the Flare Stopper Diet better than Commercial Enteral Nutrition

1. **Better Taste**: Commercial formulas are not palatable to some patients. As I said before, many patients find the taste of canned and powdered drinks disgusting, and they simply refuse to drink it for weeks in a row. Conversely, The Flare Stopper Diet is easy to digest, tastes good, and allows patients to stay on a liquid diet for extended periods of time. Plus, it's safe, easy to prepare, and inexpensive.

2. **Better Ingredients**: Commercial formulas contain ingredients that may trigger more bloating, abdominal pain, and diarrhea in some IBD patients. These are the gut offenders: milk, soy, sugar, thickeners like carrageenan, artificial flavors, artificial sweeteners, synthetic dye, and GMO ingredients (dextrose, maltodextrin, soy lecithin, corn oil, soybean oil). Whereas The Flare Stopper Diet can be prepared at home with high quality organic ingredients, without harmful additives and possible allergens like milk, soy, sugar, etc.

3. **Live vs Dead food**: The Flare Stopper Diet supercharges your body with live enzymes, bioavailable vitamins/minerals, and easy to digest nutrients, ensuring healing from inside out. You will set in motion a process of total body revitalization.

   On the contrary, commercial formulas have NO live enzymes, and are made in a highly processed form that is void of the energy and nutritional content of living food. Organic, whole foods in The Flare Stopper Diet help lower GI inflammation, support the growth of beneficial bacteria, and improve the integrity of the intestinal barrier.

The Flare Stopper Diet (Initial Phase)

This diet helps you detoxify and cleanse your body out from most known food allergens and gut irritants such as dairy (lactose, casein), all grains (especially gluten), fructose, sucrose, corn syrup, processed foods, GMO foods/ingredients, trans fats, refined oils, artificial flavors/ colors, preservatives, gums and thickeners.

The Flare Stopper Diet is divided in 2 stages: initial and transitional. Initial phase should be done for 14 days. Transitional phase should be done for 7 days.

Gut Healing Beverages You Can Drink during Initial Phase

- Alkaline Water (1 cups daily)
- Colon Cleansing Drink (2 cups daily)
- Medicinal Clay Drink™ (3 cups daily)
- Intestinal Comfort Tea™ (3 cups daily)
- Galina's Electrolyte Drink (4-6 cups/day)
- Organic flaxseed tea or CloroFlax Tea (3 cups daily)
- Organic fresh diluted vegetable juice (4 cups/day)
- GelaTannic Drink (Gelatin or Hydrolyzed Collagen mixed with Black tea 2-3 cups daily)

Soups You can eat during Initial Phase

Soups are an important part of The Flare Stopper Diet. They offer hot, delicious, easy to digest meals full of vitamins and minerals. Two soups recommended in this phase are truly gut comfort food.

- Pumpkin/Butternut Squash Soup (2 bowls/day)
- Homemade Chicken Soup (2 bowls/day)

Alkaline Water

If you are in a flare, your body is acidic. Did you know that tap water is usually acidic? You do not need more acidity when you are experiencing a flare, which is an overall acidic condition.

Reducing acidity is the key to reducing inflammation. Therefore, drinking NATURALLY alkaline water (pH 7.5-9) is essential to your quick recovery because it improves the overall alkalinity of the body; plus, it contains more minerals.

Drinking Alkaline Water Lowers Blood Viscosity

A 2016 study with 100 adults found that drinking alkaline water lowers blood viscosity when compared to drinking standard purified water. Your blood viscosity is an indicator of how well blood flows through the blood vessels. Reduced blood viscosity with the help of alkaline water will result in better oxygen delivery to your organs and tissues, which will speed up your recovery.[13]

If you want alkaline water, look for water sourced from natural springs. Do NOT use municipal (tap) water that is purified.

Examples of alkaline water:

- Volvic - pH 7.5
- Vittel - pH 7.5
- Fiji - pH 7.8
- Acqua Panna (Italy spring water) - pH 8.2
- Icelandic Glacial (Iceland spring water) - pH 8.4
- Iceland Pure Spring water - pH 8.8

Examples of purified tap water with acidic pH (do not use these):

- Dasani - pH 4
- Aquafina - pH 5
- Deja Blue - pH 6.2

Electrolytes and Water

What are electrolytes and why we need them

Electrolytes are minerals that have an electrical charge. They facilitate muscle contractions, transmit nerve signals, and keep a healthy blood pH in the normal range of 7.3-7.4. Without electrolytes your heart will stop beating, your blood will not clot, and your new tissue will not be built. So, we absolutely need electrolytes to survive.

When you have vomiting or diarrhea, you lose electrolytes. Also, you lose electrolytes when you sweat, especially if you have a fever. So, people with IBD during a flare may experience fever, vomiting and diarrhea, so they would need more electrolytes than a healthy person. The fluids together with electrolytes must be replaced to prevent dehydration and for normal body functions.

Here are the most important electrolytes:

Sodium (Na+) is vital to keep fluids around the cell in a balance. With chronic diarrhea during colitis and Crohn's flares, you can experience loss of sodium called hyponatremia (low blood sodium) which can cause fatigue, muscle cramps, nausea, and vomiting.

Potassium (K+) is vital for normal function of nerve and muscle cells. Going to the bathroom multiple times a day can trigger hypokalemia (low blood potassium). Symptoms of hypokalemia include heart palpitations, muscle spasms, or damage and numbness. If you have severe hypokalemia, you must be hospitalized and given potassium intravenously.

Bicarbonate or baking soda is a combination of sodium ions (Na) and bicarbonate ions (HCO3). Bicarbonate is a base that neutralizes acids in the blood. Severe diarrhea can cause metabolic acidosis, which is an acid-base disorder. When untreated, it can be life threatening. That is why we should add pure baking soda to our electrolyte drink - soda is a highly alkaline compound.

Commercial Electrolyte Drinks

When you are in a flare, or experiencing chronic diarrhea, you are losing life-sustaining electrolytes at an alarming rate. That is why doctors recommend commercial electrolyte drinks (such as Gatorade for adults or Pedialyte for children) - to prevent dehydration and life–threatening electrolyte imbalance. On the surface, it sounds good and should resolve the problem. Right?

Well, this may be true for some, but NOT for some people with ulcerative colitis and Crohn's disease. So, what is the problem? The problem is twofold:

Problem #1 Harmful ingredients:

An excessive amount of refined sugars (mostly GMO) are added in the form of dextrose and sucrose syrup. You'll also find artificial colors, artificial sweeteners, and preservatives (citric acid, mostly GMO derived). Maybe this sounds familiar. See for yourself the list of ingredients for Gatorade and Pedialyte:

Gatorade Ingredients: Water, Sucrose Syrup, Glucose-Fructose Syrup, Citric Acid, Natural Grape Flavor, Salt, Sodium Citrate, Monopotassium Phosphate, Red 40, Blue 1.

Pedialyte Ingredients: Water, Dextrose. Less than 2% of: Citric Acid, Potassium Citrate, Salt, Sodium Citrate, Natural Flavor, Sucralose, Acesulfame Potassium, Zinc Gluconate, Red 40, and Blue 1.

Remember the commercial Enteral Nutrition formulas - all these ingredients are known to irritate a sensitive gut. Do you need more irritation during your flare? I don't think so.

Problem #2 Not Enough Electrolytes

People with Inflammatory Bowel Disease need much more electrolytes than the average person, simply because they lose more.

Commercial electrolyte drinks simply don't have enough electrolytes to satisfy the increased needs of IBD patients during a flare. This conclusion has been confirmed by researchers from the University of Michigan IBD Team.[14]

This is why, I created Galina's Electrolyte Drink. It's a simple, healthy way to quickly replace the fluids and electrolytes you lose during your illness.

Galina's Electrolyte Drink is full of life-supporting minerals, free of harmful additives, and super affordable.

Galina's Electrolyte Drink Recipe

Many years ago, during my flares, I tried drinking both Gatorade and Pedialyte. However, I noticed that I felt worse after drinking them.

So, I took my time to study the reasons why. Just a short analysis of the ingredients revealed the problem. It became clear to me that commercial electrolyte drinks have way too much sugar, chemicals, and preservatives that increase gut inflammation.

How could I get the electrolytes I needed so desperately - without the downsides?

Out of necessity, I created Galina's Electrolyte Drink. This healing rehydration drink is so easy to make. It takes less than 5 minutes to prepare with ingredients you might already have at home.

Galina's Electrolyte Drink has only six ingredients: water, salt, baking soda, lemon juice, molasses, and potassium chloride.

I used molasses as a sweetener because it contains natural cane sugar that increases absorption of the sodium and potassium in this drink. Molasses also has a lower glycemic load than sugar (65 for sugar, 55 for molasses). And, unlike refined white table sugar, molasses contains high levels of iron, potassium, selenium, magnesium, calcium, and vitamin B6 - much needed for IBD patients during a flare.

Also, I recommend pink Himalayan salt because it has 84 trace minerals that bring balance and health to the body.

Ingredients:

- 1 liter of water (about 32 ounces or 4 cups)
- Juice of 1 organic lemon
- 1 teaspoon of organic unsulfured blackstrap molasses
- ½ teaspoon of Himalayan salt
- ½ teaspoon of baking soda
- ¼ teaspoon of potassium chloride

Directions:

1. In a pot, heat ½ cup of water until hot.
2. Add molasses, salt, and baking soda. Stir well until fully dissolved.
3. Add 3.5 cups of filtered, boiled, room temperature water.
4. Add lemon juice. Mix well.
5. If you are experiencing diarrhea, drink 1 cup of Galina's Electrolyte Drink every 1-2 hours at room temperature.
6. When your BMs (bowel movements) normalize, and frequency goes down to 2 BMs a day, decrease the amount of electrolyte drink to 2-3 cups a day for another week.
7. Store the leftover drink in mason jars or glass bottles. Drink it warm or at room temperature.

Homemade Chicken Soup (Grandma's Recipe)

Chicken broth can be part of a "clear liquid diet", which is often prescribed before or after surgery, or for patients with serious digestive problems.

Why is the word "clear" so important? Because pieces of food floating in the chicken broth can irritate your gut. "Clear" means you can see through the liquid, and after you drink it, it will not leave any food residue in your intestines.

I find that chicken broth is more effective in restoring your gut health than any man-made supplement you can buy in a health food store.

Why should you bother making your own chicken broth?

If you want the real deal in giving your body gut-restoring nutrients, you have to make it yourself. Most commercially prepared broths are made with low quality, cheap ingredients, high temperature, and various toxic additives like the MSG and meat flavors found in bouillon cubes. And making your own chicken broth is quite simple. My son could follow the recipe to make it when he was just 10 years old.

Chicken soup is not called "Jewish penicillin" for nothing. A recent study of chicken broth was done by the University of Nebraska Medical Center. Researchers found that chicken stock made according to "Grandma's recipe" (chicken, onion, sweet potatoes, parsnips, turnips, carrots, celery stems, parsley, salt and pepper) has an anti-inflammatory effect, and may improve rehydration status, and provide nutrition and physical comfort to the body.[15]

This hearty, flavorful chicken soup is truly the ultimate gut comfort food. If you are drinking broth only, the rest of the soup (chicken and veggies) can be enjoyed by other members of your family. Organic veggies and organic chicken are highly recommended.

Ingredients:

- 1 gallon of filtered water (4 quarts)
- 1 organic whole chicken, washed and cut into 8 pieces
- 5 carrots, sliced in half lengthwise
- 5 stalks of celery, sliced in half
- 1 parsley root, sliced in half
- 1 large onion, sliced in 4 pieces
- 1 leek, sliced in half and chopped
- 7 cloves of garlic, peeled and crushed
- 1 teaspoon of fresh dill
- 1 Tablespoon of coarse sea salt
- 1 dash of red cayenne pepper
- 1 dash of freshly ground black pepper

Directions:

1. Bring water to a boil. Add chicken pieces.
2. Lower heat from boiling, until at a simmer. Let simmer for 30 minutes total. Every 5 minutes for the first 20 minutes, skim off the foam (aka "scum"). I like to remove foam because if you don't, your broth may become cloudy. I prefer clear broth.
3. Add all the vegetables, and simmer for another 2 hours. Continue skimming off the foam every 30 minutes.
4. Turn off the heat. Season with salt, cayenne and black pepper, and red pepper. Stir well. Let stand for 10 minutes.
5. Strain the broth. Discard all the vegetables.
6. Serve hot in beautiful bowls!

Pumpkin/Butternut Squash Soup Recipe

People with IBD typically experience deficiency in vitamin A and potassium, especially during diarrhea and intestinal inflammation. Don't even think of taking mega doses of vitamin A and potassium supplements - that can further irritate your gut during a flare.

How do you replenish lost Vitamin A and potassium safely with food?

Use homemade butternut soup for your gut rescue. Did you know that one cup of cooked, mashed butternut squash (about 1 bowl of soup) provides an astonishing amount of vitamin A? It provides 12,231 IU of vitamin A, which is 245% of the recommended daily value. It also gives you 582 mg of potassium, which is about 30% more than the amount available in one banana.

That is why I love this rich, thick soup. It takes just 15 minutes to prepare, and this creamy, soothing wonder food is enjoyed by both kids and adults.

You will love this rich, thick, gut-nourishing, warm gift of nature. It's an integral part of the program.

Ingredients:

- 3 cups of water
- Medium-size butternut squash, about 2 pounds (peeled, seeded and sliced)
- 1 Tablespoon organic extra virgin coconut oil or organic extra virgin olive oil
- ¼ tsp of turmeric powder
- Pinch of black pepper
- Sea salt to taste

Directions:

1. Bring water to boil. Add butternut squash.
2. Turn down heat, & simmer for 15-20 minutes.
3. Add oil, turmeric powder, black pepper, and sea salt.
4. Using an immersion blender, blend for 30 seconds or until smooth. If using a blender, follow blender's instructions for blending hot soup (using a blender with too much steaming hot liquid may cause the top to pop off).
5. Serve hot and enjoy.

Fresh Vegetable Juices

Fresh, raw juice provides a colossal array of phytonutrients with anti-inflammatory activity which has a tremendous healing effect on the digestive organs and entire body of malnourished IBD patients. The process of juicing separates fiber from liquid matter in fruits and vegetables, so nutrients are absorbed very quickly into your blood. Raw vegetable juices are highly alkaline food that may regulate your body's pH.

According to Ray C. Wunderlich, M.D. and Carson Wade (a well-known medical reporter):

> *"The nutritional benefits of raw juices are most evident in those persons who are nutrient-deprived. The accumulated impact of convenience eating has taken its toll, and excessive use of antibiotics, birth control pills and corticosteroid drugs, along with the excessive consumption of fats, salt, sugar, coated and overcooked foods and undesirable food additives are associated with an epidemic of functional gastroenteropathy- faulty bowel function.*
>
> *Raw juice therapy can produce such consistent beneficial effects. Raw juice makes almost no demand upon digestive organs struggling with a daily load of cooked and often devitalized junk foods. Whole food requires hours of gut work for digestion. So, raw juices save the gut and tend to restore body vitality. With the use of richly concentrated juices, a powerhouse of nutrients as created by Nature and untouched by processing, your immune system will be strengthened and invigorated to resist and cast out hurtful invaders and shield you against ill health. Look younger, live longer and extend the prime of life with the sparkling freshness of raw juices! They are truly the elixir of life!"* [16]

I recommend juicing mostly whole, raw, organic vegetables. I do not recommend fruit juices because fruit juices contain a lot of sugar, which can initiate a rapid rise in blood glucose and increased growth in intestinal yeast/Candida. Therefore, pure fruit juices should be avoided. However, lemons can be added to vegetable juice for extra vitamin C kick and flavor.

How Juice Fasting Saved My Life

Back in 1989, a famous iridologist in Canada told me that I must do juice fasting and colonics to stop one of my worst UC flares. I thought she was crazy, and that I would die without eating any solid food for 3 weeks. I was merely 109 pounds - a pale, skinny shadow of my normal self (my normal weight was about 135 pounds).

However, I decided to give juice fasting a try. And after my first few days on the juice fast, I felt great, and my energy level was high. I realized that juice fasting is a must for anyone who desires to recover from a serious illness like ulcerative colitis. After I had completed my 3-week vegetable juicing program with other nutritional supplements and medicinal enemas, my profuse bleeding, mucus, and diarrhea stopped.

I could finally lead a normal life. I felt like I was on the top of the world. For the first time in 8 years, I was in control of my own destiny. I understood that I could be well without using harmful drugs and painful surgeries.

Fasting Accelerates Healing in IBD

Two authorities on fasting, Dr. Joel Furman (author of the book *Fasting and Eating to Health*) and Dr. Herbert Sheldon (author of the book *Fasting Can Save Your Life*), state that fasting allows the body to recover from serious illness. Also, fasting can accelerate healing of the digestive tract in patients with ulcerative colitis and Crohn's disease.

Dr. Furman's opinion is that "fasting enables long time disease sufferers to unchain themselves from their multiple toxic drugs and even eliminate the need for surgery, which was recommended to some of them as their only solution." [17]

Warning: Bottled Juice is Dead

We are all very busy people. Right? Well, I know that I am, and I suspect that you are, too. So, you may ask: "Why do I need to bother preparing my own juice if I can buy the same juice in a bottle?"

Well, the answer is simple: IT IS NOT THE SAME JUICE. The truth is that any bottled, canned, or frozen juice must be pasteurized. Pasteurization heats the product to a high temperature in order to prevent spoilage by killing bacteria, viruses, molds, and yeast. However, this heating has a largely negative effect. Along with bad bacteria, pasteurization kills live enzymes and antioxidants. So, anytime you drink pasteurized, canned, or bottled juice, you are depriving your body of compounds that it needs to heal.

The answer is simple: We MUST drink fresh squeezed juice to achieve maximum benefit. To maximize the intake of live enzymes and vitamins, consume the juice no later than 5 minutes after the squeeze. When you squeeze and drink immediately, you are consuming a very powerful substance that is both extremely healing and easy to digest – an almost perfect food for people with digestive disorders.

Why Raw Vegetable Juicing Works so well for IBD

1. Individuals with digestive diseases, especially colitis and Crohn's, have difficulty digesting and absorbing nutrients from solid foods. Juicing is a good solution for these patients because it removes hard to digest insoluble fiber. It also allows the digestive system to easily absorb nutrients, enzymes, vitamins, and minerals, which are vital for colon healing and

overall health. Eight ounces of freshly squeezed juice packs in the vitamin content of one pound of raw vegetables.

2. You can prepare gut healing raw juice at home in minutes with the most basic juicer. Raw juice has an abundant supply of live enzymes, so vital to every organ in our body. Cooked food is void of raw enzymes because heating above 130°F temperature destroys life-giving enzymes. Enzymes are the very elements that stimulate your body's healing, regenerate organs, and enhance healthy digestion and absorption of food.
3. During an IBD flare, you do not want to overwhelm your digestive system with extra work. Raw juices help your body digest and absorb all healing nutrients quickly and easily, in a matter of minutes, thus allowing the inflamed gut to rest and heal. Raw, live juice is so soothing for ulcers because it has a unique concentration of vitamins, minerals, carbohydrates, proteins, and trace minerals.
4. Your GI tract gets a break from working on digesting solid foods, which are often highly processed, overcooked, GMO altered, and full of chemicals, preservatives, and artificial dyes.
5. Fresh vegetable juices are a powerhouse of nutrients that support the body in rebuilding healthy intestines, reducing inflammation, calming down the overactive immune system, regaining energy, and initiating healing of your organs and tissues.

Vegetable Juicing: Step-by-Step Method

Are you intimidated by juicing? Not sure where to start? That's okay, I wasn't born knowing how to juice, either! Here's a handy little guide to follow.

Important: cleanliness, freshness, and organic origin of all vegetables must be emphasized to maximize the healing power of raw juice. This important rule is especially essential when it comes to conditions like colitis and Crohn's disease. Use of organic vegetables is highly recommended, so you can avoid consuming toxic pesticides sprayed on conventional produce. By drinking vegetable juices, you purify your blood, initiate an alkaline reaction in your body and feed your body with nutrients and live enzymes. So, it is WIN, WIN, WIN for your body. Enjoy!

Juicers

First, get yourself a good, reliable juicer. Although you may have your own preference, let me share my own experience with juicers. I have 2 juicers: a Breville, which I use for juicing vegetables (carrots, beets, celery, etc.) and a Slowstar which I use for green leaves. I like the Breville because I can juice whole vegetables without pre-cutting them. Cleaning it is quick and easy. I've had mine for 10 years, and I've used it almost every day. The Slowstar takes a longer time to clean; that is why I juice the green leaves and freeze extra juice to save on clean-up time.

You can find links to these juicers at:
http://knowyourgut.com/resources/

What you should juice

Attention: during this program, juice only what is recommended. If you don't tolerate any of the vegetable juices described below, just discontinue adding this problematic vegetable to your juice regimen.

Carrots: Carrot juice is one of the best natural sources of concentrated vitamin A and beta carotene (a precursor to the active form of vitamin A). Carrot juice can perform miracles, especially for those who are fighting inflammation and healing wounds.

Celery: Celery juice is rich in magnesium, organic sodium, silicon, vitamin A, and iron. Celery juice has a cooling effect on an inflamed gut - great for anyone with ulcerative colitis and Crohn's disease. Furthermore, celery provides organic, easy to absorb calcium that helps IBD patients strengthen their bones and protect against osteoporosis.

Beets: Beetroot juice is a natural blood builder and detoxifier. For people with IBD these properties are especially important since beet juice provides lots of iron and helps regenerate red blood cells. All these factors are important for treating anemia in IBD. Moreover, thanks to the betalain compound in beets, beet juice can cleanse the body of toxins, waste, and heavy metals. Also, betalain in beet juice supports formation of glutathione, an important antioxidant that helps fight cellular damage.

You might be surprised to learn that IBD medications, such as Sulfasalazine and Methotrexate, interfere with production of B vitamin (folate) in the human body. Drinking beet juice will nourish your body with natural folate. Just one 8 oz. glass of fresh beet juice provides 294 milligrams of natural B vitamin (folate).

Greens (Parsley, Kale, Romaine Lettuce): All greens have one thing in common - chlorophyll (the green pigment that gives vegetables their green color).

What is so special about chlorophyll? Chlorophyll is a great oxygenator and blood builder. When taken internally, it delivers oxygen to tissues and increases the number of red blood cells. This can help improve hemoglobin levels in IBD patients with anemia. Oxygen deprivation is one of the major causes of the IBD disease process. Chlorophyll increases oxygen delivery to organs and tissues, which helps heal the inflamed intestinal lining and suppress pathogenic organisms in the gut. Therefore, adding some chlorophyll-rich green juice to your vegetable juice is crucial for regaining gut health quickly.

Lemon: Lemon is a wonderful fruit that helps you alkalize and detoxify your body. It also provides a boost of vitamin C, potassium, magnesium, and calcium. Adding lemon juice to your electrolyte drink is a must for rehydration and detoxification of your body.

Do's & Don'ts of Juicing

- NO FRUITS ARE ALLOWED for juicing, except lemons.
- Use organic produce only, to avoid pesticides and insecticides.

- Disinfect vegetables after peeling and prior to juicing.
- Dilute the juice 50% with pure boiled water, at a lukewarm temperature.

Juicing Recipes

Ingredients vary depending on the kind of juice you'd like to make. Here are three different recipes. You can use one or all three, depending on your preference.

Ingredients:

- **Clean Green Power:** 3 ribs of celery, romaine lettuce, ½ cup parsley, ½ lemon (peeled).
- **Blood Builder:** 3 peeled carrots, 1 small, peeled beet, 3 celery stalks, 2 kale leaves, ½ bunch of parsley
- **Immune Booster:** 4 peeled carrots, 4 ribs of celery, 1 peeled lemon, 1 peeled beet, ½" peeled fresh turmeric, 2 peeled cloves of garlic

When to drink:

During a flare, drink 1 cup of juice every 3 hours (total of 4-5 cups daily) diluted 50% with filtered, boiled, cooled water. Supplement with oil of your choice such as fish oil or organic flaxseed oil.

Directions:

1. Wash your hands for 20-25 seconds with soap and water.
2. Wash, scrub, and peel all vegetables thoroughly.
3. Prepare disinfection solution: in a large pot full of 1 gallon of filtered, boiled, cooled water, add ¼ cup or 4 tablespoons of 3% hydrogen peroxide. Use this disinfection solution to kill off possible E. coli and other pathogenic microorganisms that may be present on the surface of the vegetables.

4. Place the vegetables in the disinfection solution. Keep them there for 10 minutes.
5. Remove vegetables from the disinfection solution and drain them in a colander. Then, place your disinfected vegetables in another large pot full of 1 gallon of filtered, boiled, cooled water. Keep them there for a few minutes to remove the remaining peroxide. Then, drain vegetables again in a colander.
6. Now, juice your vegetables. After juicing:
7. **Dilute.** For better absorption, the raw juice should be diluted with filtered, boiled, cooled water in a ratio of 50% juice + 50% water. To suit your taste, you can use less water for dilution.
8. **Supplement with oil.** For better absorption of fat-soluble vitamins (vitamin A and vitamin K) in your juice, drink 1 teaspoon of fish oil or organic flaxseed oil with your juice. Don't add it to the juice, just drink it directly from the teaspoon.
9. **Drink immediately.** Since vitamins and enzymes in fresh juice degrade quickly, try drinking your fresh juice within 5 minutes of juicing to maximize its potency and healing power.

   After you are done, wash your juicer, knives, and boards with soap and hot water. Let them air dry. Repeat the process the next day.

Can you bulk prepare juice?

Ideally, raw, live juices should be prepared fresh each time before using. However, if you don't have the energy to clean your juicer a few times a day, you can juice your day's supply in the morning and store your juice in the fridge in a covered glass container, and use it throughout the day. Ideally, for maximum nutritional benefit, plan to drink your juice right after it's been squeezed.

Flaxseed Tea Recipe

Flaxseed tea can work wonders for inflamed, bleeding bowels. It gently lubricates the irritated inner lining of the colon and heals intestinal ulcers. It works well for IBD because it calms the irritated gut. Flaxseed is a perfect demulcent, which is a substance that relieves pain and reduces inflammation of the mucous membrane. It literally coats the inner mucosa of your intestines.

Why I created ChloroFlax Tea Recipe

For years, I suffered from intestinal inflammation, hemorrhoids, and bleeding. I tried everything to soothe my pain, including:

- Creams (Preparation H, etc.)
- Foams (Proctofoam HC cortisone cream, etc.)
- Suppositories (Mumiyo, a natural European suppository, etc.)
- Hemorrhoidal Pads (Witch Hazel Medicated)

Nothing worked! I was full of despair.

One day, I came across an old Russian book with tons of folk remedies. It recommended flaxseed tea for reducing bowel inflammation. I drank flaxseed tea for a week and felt somewhat better. Then, I read an article saying chlorophyll heals ulcers and wounds. So, I started drinking chlorophyll a few times a day. Eventually I got tired of drinking so much liquid. I decided to mix the two, and voila! My ChloroFlax recipe was born.

I drank my new ChloroFlax tea for a week, and my bleeding and spasms diminished. However, I still had soreness and inflammation in my rectum. So, I decided to go to the next level. In addition to drinking ChloroFlax tea 2-3 times a day before meals, I started doing retention enemas with ChloroFlax tea at night. Together with all the other natural treatments, this recipe worked like a charm and my bleeding stopped in two weeks. My butt was no longer a pain in the ass (pun intended).

Flaxseed Tea Recipe

This flaxseed tea has a jelly-like consistency. I know it's slimy and gooey, so it might take some getting used to… but it's exactly what your body needs to start healing! You also have the option to add chlorophyll, for a double dose of goodness.

Ingredients & Supplies:

- 1 steel or enamel pot with a lid
- 3.5 cups of boiling water
- 2 Tablespoons of whole, organic flax seeds

When to drink:

- Drink 1 cup of tea, 3 times a day, 30 minutes before meals.
- For best results, drink the flaxseed tea for at least 7 weeks.

Directions:

1. Boil 3.5 cups of water.
2. Add flaxseed to boiling water. Cover with a lid. Turn flame down to low, and simmer for 15 minutes.
3. Turn off flame, & steep (covered with a lid) for another 30 minutes.
4. Strain flaxseed tea through a strainer to separate seeds from liquid. Discard the seeds.
5. Let the tea cool down until it's at body temperature, around 98°F / 37°C.
6. Drink 1 cup of flaxseed tea.
7. Refrigerate the remaining 2 cups in a glass mason jar.

8. When you're ready to drink the second and third cup, warm 1 cup of tea on the stove until it's around body temperature. (Do not use the microwave. Do not boil. Do not dilute.)

ChloroFlax Tea Recipe

This variation of Flaxseed Tea adds chlorophyll. Make sure you use organic chlorophyll. It's best to add the chlorophyll to the lukewarm tea right before you drink it. Do not add chlorophyll to hot tea.

Ingredients:

- Flaxseed Tea (recipe above)
- 6 Tablespoons of liquid, organic chlorophyll

Directions:

1. Follow the recipe above for Flaxseed Tea.
2. Warm Flaxseed Tea until it's at body temperature, around 98°F / 37°C. Do not boil.
3. Add 2 Tablespoons of chlorophyll to 1 cup of tea.
4. Drink immediately.

Hydrolyzed Collagen

What is Hydrolyzed Collagen?

Hydrolyzed collagen is a protein powder that is easy to digest because it's broken down into amino acids. These intact amino acids are used by our body as the building blocks of new collagen. Collagen is the main component of connective tissue that provides structure, elasticity, and firmness to skin, tendons, muscles, ligaments, teeth, and bones. Hydrolyzed collagen means that enzymes were added to the collagen (protein) to break it down into easy to absorb food.

Collagen is high in the amino acid glycine, which according to animal studies can inhibit TNF (Tumor Necrosis Factor), aka TNF-alpha (a protein produced by white blood cells that regulate the immune response).[18]

What does TNF have to do with IBD?

According to Dr. Prianka Chugh and Amber J. Tresca, "TNF is found in higher amounts in people with Crohn's disease than in people who do not have Crohn's disease. TNF is also found, to a lesser degree, in the stool of people who have ulcerative colitis. Because of this association, it is apparent that TNF plays a role in the development and/or continuing Crohn's disease and ulcerative colitis."[19]

Do you remember that anti-TNF drugs are used to treat inflammation in IBD?

These drugs work by "targeting the TNF protein and binding it. When the protein is bound, it is not able to produce inflammation."[19]

Studies demonstrate that a simple amino acid, glycine, can inhibit TNF protein. Did you know that collagen is high in glycine? That's right. Supplementing with collagen that is naturally high in gut-healing glycine can result in lower intestinal inflammation minus the side effects of TNF drugs.[18]

That's why adding collagen during the program is essential; it helps to reduce IBD symptoms, lower intestinal inflammation, and promote integrity of the intestinal lining.

What Hydrolyzed Collagen can do for you

Hydrolyzed collagen can:

- Decrease inflammation and joint pain
- Help maintain healthy, strong bones and joints
- Support a healthy gut lining and normal intestinal permeability

For the best quality, I use collagen made from grass-fed, pasture-raised cows, non-GMO, gluten-free, and kosher.

If a collagen supplement has a strange taste and brownish color, it's probably lower in quality. If you cannot buy hydrolyzed collagen, use plain gelatin instead. I recommend "Great Lakes Unflavored Beef Gelatin", considered the highest quality of pure, unflavored, edible gelatin.

Two Ways to Take Hydrolyzed Collagen:

1. Drink 1 scoop mixed with water, 2 times a day, or
2. Use it as part of Gelatin + Tannic acid drink & drink it 2-3 times a day.

Stop Diarrhea Fast with Gelatin and Tannic Acid (from Black Tea)

Years ago, by pure experimentation, I used a mixture of gelatin and black tea trying to stop my diarrhea. I knew that black tea is high in tannic acid (which has an antidiarrheal effect), and gelatin can help firm up stool. Both ingredients are cheap and widely available. So, I experimented mixing gelatin with black tea more than 25 years ago. I drank it when I had profuse diarrhea during my flares. Here are some studies that support these items as being beneficial to gut health.

Russian scientists conducted animal studies with gelatin. They observed that feeding gelatin to rats helps to protect their intestinal lining from damage caused by alcohol.[20]

Scientists from the University of Catania, Italy, evaluated the anti-inflammatory activity of gelatin tannate in human intestinal cells during inflammation.

So, what is gelatin tannate? It's a simple mixture of tannic acid and gelatin that can reduce intestinal inflammation by decreasing the release of cytokines (special molecules that regulate immunity).

Tannic acid is an antioxidant compound that has antibacterial and astringent properties. It has been effective in the treatment of diarrhea caused by foodborne pathogens such as E. coli and Listeria.

Gelatin, when made properly, is a pure natural protein that has no odor or flavor. It contains about 90% collagen protein, 1%–2% mineral salts, and the rest is water.

Researchers in this Italian study concluded that a mixture of gelatin and tannic acid has antibacterial, astringent, and antioxidant properties. And this powerful combination "could be used not only for its antidiarrheal effects, but also for the treatment of intestinal disorders such as inflammatory bowel conditions." Finally, the gelatin and tannic acid combo has no toxic effect on the gut when compared to "conventional antibiotics that can contribute to the development of resistance and dysbacteriosis."[21]

Later on, I began using hydrolyzed collagen instead of gelatin because it's easier to dissolve in warm tea.

Recipe for Gelatin + Tannic Acid Drink

Ingredients:

- 1 cup (8 oz) of hot boiling water
- ½ teaspoon loose organic black tea
- 1-2 Tablespoons of Hydrolyzed Collagen or Plain Gelatin

Directions:

1. Bring filtered water to a full boil.
2. Put ½ teaspoon loose organic black tea into a large cup or French press.
3. Add 1 cup of hot water and brew for 5-10 minutes.
4. After the tea is fully brewed, strain the tea leaves.
5. Pour the strained tea into a large mug.

6. Add 1-2 Tablespoons of collagen to tea. Mix well until fully dissolved.
7. Drink warm, 2 times a day. Enjoy your gut healing beverage!

Organic Black Tea Brewing Recipe

1. Bring filtered water to a full boil.
2. Measure your tea leaves. Use 1 teaspoon of tea leaves for 8 ounces of water.
3. Put your tea leaves in a French press or teapot and pour boiling water directly over the tea leaves.
4. Allow the tea to steep for 5-10 minutes. Long brewing aids release of tannins, which are very helpful at times of abdominal distress and diarrhea.

Organic Green Tea Brewing Recipe

1. Bring filtered water to a full boil.
2. Measure your tea leaves. Use 1 teaspoon of tea leaves for 8 ounces of water.
3. Please put your loose tea leaves in a French press or teapot, and pour boiling water directly over the tea leaves.
4. Allow the tea to steep for 3-5 minutes.

Important Comment:

I recommend loose leaf tea. In my opinion, loose leaf tea is good for you because it's a higher-grade tea, which retains more antioxidants and anti-inflammatory compounds. You'll find that when you open most tea bags, the tea inside is finely chopped, which promotes oxidation of tea leaves, making their benefits less potent. Moreover, most tea bags are bleached with chemicals which leach into your tea while it's brewing in hot water. So, in conclusion, use loose leaf tea, and no tea bags.

Transitional Diet

The goal of the Transitional Diet is to be the bridge, a transition from a liquid diet to a solid food diet. This transition must be done slowly.

It is very dangerous to start eating solid foods right after eating full liquid diet!

Do not eat solid foods right after a prolonged liquid diet. If you decide to ignore this rule and start eating solid foods right away, you will erase the benefits of your liquid diet. A too-quick reintroduction of solid foods can get you sick for days with stomach pain, bloating, nausea, diarrhea, or constipation.

Duration: The general rule is that the length of a transition diet should be at least 50% of the length of your liquid diet. For example, if your liquid diet lasted 14 days, the transition diet should last for at least 7 days.

Once again, do not cut the transition diet short!

You have just completed your initial diet, which jump-started your healing. Do not get impatient! The transitional diet is as important as initial diet for accelerated gut healing.

Gut Healing Beverages You can Drink during Transitional Phase

It's a fact - water is the best drink if you want to stay hydrated. That includes hot water with lemon, spring water, and mineral water. But if you also want to boost your immune system, detoxify your body and soothe your digestive system, give the following beverages a try.

- Golden milk (1 cup daily)
- Bone broth (2 cups daily)
- Alkaline Water (1-2 cup daily)

- Intestinal Comfort Tea™ (3 cups daily)
- Galina's Electrolyte Drink (2-4 cups/day)
- Organic flaxseed tea or CloroFlax Tea (3 cups daily)
- Fresh, raw vegetable juices (undiluted, up to 4 cups/day)
- Hydrolyzed Collagen drink (mixed with water or almond milk, 1 cup daily)
- Homemade almond milk (or any other nut you are not allergic to, up to 2 cups daily)

Soups You can Eat during Transitional Phase

Soups are an important part of The Flare Stopper Diet. They offer hot, delicious, easy to digest flavorful meals. These soups are rich in antioxidants and soluble fiber that boost the immune system and aid digestion.

- Blood building soup
- Pumpkin/Butternut Squash Soup
- Chicken soup with boiled carrots and zucchini (blended into a puree)

The following is a description and recipes of the added food items allowed for transitional phase diet.

Golden Milk Recipe

If you haven't tried Golden Milk, then now is the time! This soothing, delicious drink is a perfect beverage when you are feeling weak or recovering from an illness.

Both turmeric herb and ginger root that are used in this recipe have numerous benefits: they can reduce inflammation, relieve pain and support healthy immune response. By adding black pepper and coconut oil you enhance absorption and bioavailability of turmeric. You can enjoy this heavenly drink anytime to nurture your body from the inside out.

Ingredients:

- 1 teaspoon fresh peeled, grated turmeric or 1 teaspoon turmeric powder
- 1 cup of plant-based milk (almond, soy or coconut milk)
- 1 teaspoon of fresh peeled, grated ginger
- 1/2 teaspoon cinnamon
- Dash of black pepper
- 2 teaspoons of coconut oil

How to Make:

1. Heat 1 cup of plant-based milk in a saucepan.
2. Add ginger, turmeric, cinnamon, and black pepper, and stir well.
3. Turn the heat down to low and bring to a simmer. Cook for 10 minutes.
4. Turn the heat off, and add coconut oil. Stir well until oil is fully dissolved.
5. Strain the liquid directly into a mug, to remove the ginger and turmeric pieces.

Tip: After the golden milk is done, you can use a milk frother to make it creamy.

Almond Milk

Almond milk is a simple drink made from just 2 ingredients: almonds and water. It's a great vegetarian alternative to cow's milk.

Almond milk is high in protein and calcium, highly alkaline, easy to digest and simply delicious. Fresh, raw, homemade almond milk contains live enzymes with no thickeners like store bought almond milk. And it takes just 5 minutes to prepare.

Ingredients:

- 7 cups of filtered pure water
- 1 cup raw unsalted, organic almonds
- ¼ teaspoon of sea salt during soaking + ¼ teaspoon of sea salt for blending of almond milk

How to Make:

1. Put almonds in a glass/ceramic bowl, cover with water, 1/4 teaspoon of salt and soak overnight. In the morning, transfer almonds into a colander, drain the water, then rinse well.
2. Put almonds into a blender, add 7 cups of water. Let it stand for 1 minute. You will see that some almonds will float to the top. Remove them because they are rancid. Add sea salt and blend the remaining almonds well for at least 2 minutes.
3. Strain the almond milk through a fine sieve into a glass pitcher. Keep refrigerated, and use it within 2-3 days.

Bone Broth Recipe

Bone broth is a stock where meat, chicken or fish bones, vegetables, herbs, and spices are slowly cooked for 6-24 hours or longer. This way of cooking releases beneficial collagen, gelatin, 19 amino acids (including glutamine), glucosamine, chondroitin, hyaluronic acid, and minerals from the bones. This gut-soothing drink works as a healing remedy for an inflamed intestinal lining, and is effective in restoring your gut health. It can provide the following health benefits:

- Reduce inflammation
- Repair the gut lining
- Enhance overall body detoxification
- Support the health of immune system and builds muscle mass

Studies show that patients with ulcerative colitis and Crohn's disease suffer from decreased serum concentration of collagen. Collagen contains 19 amino acids that are necessary for building a healthy lining in the entire gastrointestinal tract. Therefore, you must have enough collagen in your body to rebuild new healthy tissue. Bone broth has plenty of collagen in a highly digestible form that can heal and seal the intestinal lining. Drink 2-3 servings of bone broth daily. One serving is about 8 ounces.[22]

I use the bone broth recipe below to repair the gut lining, reduce intestinal inflammation and to strengthen immunity. This healing broth contains bioavailable, easy to absorb minerals such as potassium, calcium, magnesium, phosphorus, and sulfur, as well as anti-inflammatory compounds such as chondroitin sulfate, hyaluronic acid, and glucosamine. These are often sold as man-made nutritional supplements to reduce inflammation in arthritis.

I find that this homemade bone broth is more effective in restoring your gut health than any man-made supplement you can buy in a health food store. You cannot buy this type of broth in a store; commercially prepared broth is often made with low quality, cheap ingredients, high temperature, and various additives (like MSG and artificial flavors).

Furthermore, bone broth nourishes adrenals, supports kidneys, and builds blood. Bone broth is rich in amino acids (proline, glycine, lysine) and gelatin. These compounds help in gut healing and support good digestion.

Gut healing bone broth should be made from local, organic, grass-fed animals. Use bones from any of the following animals: chickens, beef, lamb, bison, veal, and turkey. I use oxtail, marrow bones, knuckle bones, necks with some meat on them, and whole organic chicken, plus chicken feet.

Ingredients:

- 2-3 pounds of bones with some meat, or a small whole chicken & chicken feet
- 5 quarts of water

- 2 Tablespoons fresh lemon juice
- 2 onions, chopped in large pieces
- 3 carrots, chopped in 1-inch pieces
- 3 celery stalks, chopped in 1-inch pieces
- 7 garlic cloves, cut in half
- 2 bay leaves, broken in half
- Salt & pepper to taste

Directions:

1. In a pan, roast bones on both sides for 10-15 minutes, turning them over halfway. Do not deglaze the pan. Just discard the brown bits and juices from the pan, and wash the pan later.
2. In a large (8.5 quart) crockpot/slow cooker, add the roasted bones and all other ingredients. Bring to a boil.
3. Then, reduce to a simmer. During the first hour of cooking, remove the foam (aka scum) that usually floats to the top of the broth.
4. Cook for 10-12 hours. If using a slow cooker/crockpot, it can be cooked overnight.
5. Strain the stock through a fine metal mesh strainer into a pot. Let it cool.
6. Once cooled, ladle broth into glass containers or mason jars.
7. After the broth is refrigerated, you will see a layer of fat formed on the top of the broth. Remove this fat before heating the broth.
8. To prepare as a meal, add vegetables to broth and simmer for 10 minutes.
9. You can eat the broth with cooked meat and vegetables for 2-3 days.
10. Any leftover broth must be frozen.

Blood Building Soup

This flavorful, fresh-tasting soup is so easy to make. And it's loaded with nutrients that are important for people with anemia. It has dark, leafy green spinach, which provides iron, folate and vitamin C. This well spiced, delicious soup will help boost the production of red blood cells and hemoglobin in your body.

Ingredients:

- 2 quarts (8 cups) of filtered or spring water
- 1-pound organic carrots, peeled and chopped
- 5 ounces organic baby spinach
- 1 clove of garlic
- 2 teaspoons of fresh lemon juice
- 1/4 teaspoon turmeric powder
- Sea salt and cayenne pepper to taste
- Olive oil, extra virgin cold pressed (optional)

How to Make:

1. Boil 8 cups of water. Add chopped carrots and simmer for 20 minutes.
2. Add organic baby spinach and simmer for 5 more minutes
3. Add garlic and simmer for another minute. Turn the heat off.
4. Add lemon juice, sea salt, cayenne pepper and turmeric powder. Stir well.
5. Transfer the soup to a blender, and blend it for a minute.
6. Serve with olive oil that is added to hot soup. Enjoy!

Homemade Chicken Soup (Grandma's Recipe)

This hearty, flavorful chicken soup is truly the ultimate gut comfort food. Organic veggies and organic chicken are highly recommended.

Ingredients:

- 1 gallon of filtered water (4 quarts)
- 1 organic whole chicken, washed and cut into 8 pieces
- 5 carrots, sliced in half lengthwise

- 5 stalks of celery, sliced in half
- 2 parsley roots, sliced in half
- 1 large onion, sliced in 4 pieces
- 1 leek, sliced in half and chopped
- 7 cloves of garlic, peeled and crushed
- 1 teaspoon of fresh dill
- 1 Tablespoon of coarse sea salt
- 1 dash of red cayenne pepper
- 1 dash of freshly ground black pepper

Directions:

1. Bring water to a boil. Add chicken pieces.
2. Lower heat from boiling, until at a simmer. Let simmer for 30 minutes total. Every 5 minutes for the first 20 minutes, skim off the foam (aka "scum"). I like to remove foam because if you don't, your broth may become cloudy. I prefer clear broth.
3. Add all the vegetables, and simmer for another 2 hours. Continue skimming off the foam every 30 minutes.
4. Turn off the heat. Season with salt, cayenne and black pepper, and red pepper. Stir well. Let stand for 10 minutes.
5. Strain the broth. Discard all the vegetables.
6. Pour 4 cups of chicken broth into a saucepan. Add boiled carrots and 1 parsley root, and blend
7. Serve hot in beautiful bowls!

Beverages You Should Avoid

IBD patients should remain vigilant in creating a healthy balance of their gut flora. Introduction of beverages or foods containing sugar, fructose, sugar alcohols, artificial sweeteners, & citric acid can work against you by feeding harmful bacteria and fungus causing gas, bloating, and diarrhea. Therefore, I recommend avoiding the following beverages:

- Bottled or canned vegetable juices
- Bottled or canned fruit juices and fruit juice drinks

- Commercial apple cider and lemonade
- Bottled iced tea (even organic, unsweetened)
- Carbonated Drinks and Beverages
- Decaffeinated tea and coffee
- Electrolyte replacement drinks (including electrolyte tablets that are added to water)
- Commercial Energy Drinks and Cocktails
- Flavored Coffee Drinks and Flavored Water
- Kombucha tea (has sugar and may cause nausea and allergic reactions)
- Ice cream milkshakes and Sweetened Yogurt Drinks
- Muscle Milks and Meal Replacement shakes (including organic brands)
- Soda (regular, diet and made with stevia)
- Sweetened, commercial plant milk (almond, oatmeal, rice, hazelnut, etc.)

Bottled/Boxed/Canned Fruit and Vegetable Juices and Drinks

All bottled juices are pasteurized. Pasteurization kills live enzymes and most vitamins. You are left with a bottle of dead juice filled with lots of sugar (fructose). Some manufactures add extra sweeteners, preservatives, and colors. Also, juices tend to contain mold and cancer-causing heavy metals like arsenic and lead (like in apple juice and grape juice).

Consumer Reports tested 88 samples of apple and grape juice. They found that, "Five samples of apple juice and four of grape juice had total arsenic levels exceeding the 10-ppb federal limit for bottled and drinking water. Levels in the apple juices ranged from 1.1 to 13.9 ppb, and grape-juice levels were even higher, 5.9 to 24.7 ppb. Most of the total arsenic in our samples was inorganic, our tests showed. As for lead, about one fourth of all juice samples had levels at or above the 5-ppb limit for bottled water. The top lead level for apple juice was 13.6 ppb; for grape juice, 15.9 ppb."[23]

Therefore, I insist on using freshly prepared vegetable juice to build your blood and heal your colon.

Alcohol

Sorry, wine, beer, and adult beverage lovers. A glass of red wine and an occasional drink can be acceptable for regular folks, but for IBD patients, any alcohol, even once a week during gut healing, can have a devastating effect on their gut.

A pattern of alcohol consumption was evaluated in a a recent study of 90 patients with Crohn's and colitis. It was reported that in 75% of IBD patients, alcohol consumption either triggered a flare or aggravated their gastrointestinal symptoms.

If you have GERD in addition to IBD, alcohol should be off your menu because alcohol has been known to worsen GERD by decreasing the lower esophageal sphincter (LES) tone. This allows the stomach's contents to flow back into the esophagus causing pain, nausea, burping, heartburn, and regurgitation.

The Bottom Line: You can enjoy a healthy life without drinking alcohol! However, if you are in remission for at least 2 years, you can have a glass of red wine or champagne on special occasions a few times a year (your birthday, New Year, Christmas, etc.)[24]

I know I do. Cheers!

Conclusion

Now you've learned about The Flare Stopper Diet which will contribute to the elimination of your diarrhea, abdominal pain, and bleeding. Now you're on the way to reversing the IBD disease process and achieving true gut healing.

Next, we'll learn about supplements.

References

[1] Hunter, John. "Elemental diet and the nutritional treatment of Crohn's disease." *Gastroenterology and hepatology from bed to bench* vol. 8,1 (2015): 4-5. https://www.ncbi.nlm.nih.gov/pmc/articles/PMC4285926/

[2] Matsui, Toshiyuki et al. "Nutritional therapy for Crohn's disease in Japan." *Journal of gastroenterology* vol. 40 Suppl 16 (2005): 25-31. doi:10.1007/BF02990575 https://pubmed.ncbi.nlm.nih.gov/15902960/

[3] Yamamoto, Takayuki et al. "Enteral nutrition for the maintenance of remission in Crohn's disease: a systematic review." *European journal of gastroenterology & hepatology* vol. 22,1 (2010): 1-8. doi:10.1097/MEG.0b013e32832c788c

[4] Carla Andrade Lima et al., "Risk factors for osteoporosis in inflammatory bowel disease patients." *World J Gastrointest Pathophysiol.* 2015 Nov 15; 6(4): 210–218. Published online 2015 Nov 15. doi: 10.4291/wjgp.v6.i4.210

[5] Soo, Jason et al. "Use of exclusive enteral nutrition is just as effective as corticosteroids in newly diagnosed pediatric Crohn's disease." *Digestive diseases and sciences* vol. 58,12 (2013): 3584-91. doi:10.1007/s10620-013-2855-y https://pubmed.ncbi.nlm.nih.gov/24026403/

[6] https://www.healio.com/gastroenterology/inflammatory-bowel-disease/news/online/%7Be0ce6a90-ab8d-4029-ad35-482c66c2b870%7D/exclusive-enteral-nutrition-effective-as-steroids-for-pediatric-crohns

[7] O'Moráin, C et al. "Elemental diet as primary treatment of acute Crohn's disease: a controlled trial." *British medical journal* (Clinical research ed.) vol. 288,6434 (1984): 1859-62. doi:10.1136/bmj.288.6434.1859 https://www.ncbi.nlm.nih.gov/pmc/articles/PMC1441790/

[8] Levine, Arie et al. "Consensus and controversy in the management of pediatric Crohn disease: an international survey." *Journal of pediatric gastroenterology and nutrition* vol. 36,4 (2003): 464-9. doi:10.1097/00005176-200304000-00008 https://pubmed.ncbi.nlm.nih.gov/12658036/

[9] http://digestivemedicalsolutions.com/the-good-the-bad-and-the-ugly-side-of-gmos-and-their-link-to-ibd

[10] Kobylewski, S., Ph.D, Jacobson, M., Ph.D. (2010). "Food Dyes: Rainbow of Risks." *Center for Science in the Public Interest* https://cspinet.org/new/201006291.html

[11] Marcus, A J et al. "Rapid production of ulcerative disease of the colon in newly-weaned guinea-pigs by degraded carrageenan." *The Journal of pharmacy and pharmacology* vol. 41,6 (1989): 423-6. doi:10.1111/j.2042-7158.1989.tb06493.x https://pubmed.ncbi.nlm.nih.gov/2570843/

[12] Tobacman, J K. "Review of harmful gastrointestinal effects of carrageenan in animal experiments." *Environmental health perspectives* vol. 109,10 (2001): 983-94. doi:10.1289/ehp.01109983 https://www.ncbi.nlm.nih.gov/pmc/articles/PMC1242073/

[13] Weidman, J., Holsworth, R.E., Brossman, B. et al. "Effect of electrolyzed high-pH alkaline water on blood viscosity in healthy adults." *J Int Soc Sports* Nutr 13, 45 (2016). https://doi.org/10.1186/s12970-016-0153-8

[14] University of Michigan IBD Team Facebook post. Trying to rehydrate with Gatorade? January 18, 2016.

[15] Rennard, B. et al. "Chicken Soup Inhibits Neutrophil Chemotaxis In Vitro*." CHEST 2000; 118:1150 –1157

[16] Wade C., R.C. Wunderlich, M.D. (1988) *Juice Power*. Keats Publishing

[17] Dr. Furman J. (1995). *Fasting and Eating for Health*. St. Martin's Griffin

[18] Razak, Meerza Abdul et al. "Multifarious Beneficial Effect of Nonessential Amino Acid, Glycine: A Review." *Oxidative medicine and cellular longevity* vol. 2017 (2017): 1716701. doi:10.1155/2017/1716701

[19] https://www.verywellhealth.com/tumor-necrosis-factor-alpha-1942547

[20] Samonina, G et al. "Protection of gastric mucosal integrity by gelatin and simple proline-containing peptides." *Pathophysiology: the official journal of the International Society for Pathophysiology* vol. 7,1 (2000): 69-73. doi:10.1016/s0928-4680(00)00045-6

[21] Frasca, Giuseppina et al. "Gelatin tannate reduces the proinflammatory effects of lipopolysaccharide in human intestinal epithelial cells." *Clinical and experimental gastroenterology* vol. 5 (2012): 61-7. doi:10.2147/CEG.S28792

[22] Koutroubakis, I E et al. "Serum laminin and collagen IV in inflammatory bowel disease." *Journal of clinical pathology* vol. 56,11 (2003): 817-20. doi:10.1136/jcp.56.11.817

[23] http://www.consumerreports.org/cro/magazine/2012/01/arsenic-in-your-juice/index.htm

[24] Swanson, Garth R et al. "Pattern of alcohol consumption and its effect on gastrointestinal symptoms in inflammatory bowel disease." *Alcohol (Fayetteville, N.Y.)* vol. 44,3 (2010): 223-8. doi:10.1016/j.alcohol.2009.10.019
https://www.ncbi.nlm.nih.gov/pmc/articles/PMC3708696/

CHAPTER 11

Dietary Supplements

DIETARY SUPPLEMENTS CAN BE A USEFUL TOOL IN HEALING. FIRST, IT'S important to choose the correct supplements. Second, the supplements you choose need to be of high quality in order to work effectively.

In order to make these choices easier, I assembled a package of dietary supplements for my clients. It's called The Flare Stopper™ Kit for IBD. It has been designed for safe, yet powerful cleansing and detoxification of the body. It contains antimicrobial herbs, medicinal clay, anti-inflammatory essential oils, colon cleansing fiber, and activated charcoal. Most of my patients have been amazed by how quickly they could reverse the disease process and restore their normal gut functions. The Flare Stopper Kit supplements help neutralize and excrete the toxins that are stored in your body and your gut.

Although some of my clients were amazed as to how quickly they started to feel better (after being on the program for 5 to 7 days), I recommend staying on this program for at least 21 days for those with moderate cases. For those with severe cases (like my own), I had to be on the program for 30 days. Thorough cleansing is necessary to start the process of your recovery, and The Flare Stopper Kit is the tool that can help.

Warning/Disclaimer: Please note that without definite medical diagnoses and proper nutritional assessment of your medical history (labs, etc.), administration of any nutritional supplements may not be effective, or can even cause an adverse effect. Always consult with your doctor prior to taking any nutritional supplements.

The Flare Stopper Kit for IBD

I formulated The Flare Stopper Kit with the needs of IBD people in mind. The natural products in the kit, together with The Flare Stopper Diet, were designed to repair the damaged gastrointestinal mucosa, lower overall level of inflammation, and restore digestive health. After cleansing and detoxification are completed, you will experience abundance of energy and vitality, plus better absorption of vitamins and nutrients, resulting in healthy weight gain.

Note: Do not expect that you will feel great instantaneously just because you are doing a few days of cleansing. Decades of toxin accumulation must be disposed of gently and slowly. This usually takes time and lots of patience. While on the cleansing program you might experience peaks and valleys in your mood and energy. On some days, you will feel great, while on others you may feel awful. Some of these toxins get into your bloodstream and make you feel lousy. All that is a normal part of your cleansing and detoxification while your body releases toxins stored in your tissues. But The Flare Stopper Kit is designed to help your body to get rid of these toxins as soon as possible.

The Flare Stopper Kit for IBD has 11 key items:

1. Intestinal Comfort Tea™
2. Immunity G7 Formula™
3. Medicinal Clay™
4. Colon Formula™
5. Cod Liver Oil
6. Activated Charcoal
7. Bentonite
8. Psyllium Husk

9. Hydrolyzed Collagen
10. Potassium Chloride
11. Chlorophyll

You can buy The Flare Stopper Kit™ from my website: https://knowyourgut.com/products/

In addition to the instructions below, I've created videos on how to prepare Intestinal Comfort Tea, Medicinal Clay Drink and Medicinal Clay Poultice. You can follow along here: knowyourgut.com/video/.

Let's discuss each item in the Immediate Help Kit in detail.

Intestinal Comfort Tea™

What is Intestinal Comfort Tea?

Intestinal Comfort Tea was specially designed for digestive health and wellness. It's made with certified organic medicinal grade herbs, backed by science for their antibacterial, antiviral, anti-inflammatory, and pain-relieving properties.

What does Intestinal Comfort Tea do?

Herbs used in this tea were used as a treatment for 24 patients with colitis living in Bulgaria. After only 15 days of herbal treatments, 95% of colitis patients felt better: no more abdominal pain and no more diarrhea.[1]

The main ingredient in Intestinal Comfort Tea is Melissa Officinalis. This herb has been approved by the German Commission E (German Federal Health Agency) for the following:

- Abdominal pain and spasm
- Gas, bloating, and loss of appetite
- Wounds, inflammation, and tissue repair

Why don't we use tea bags for Intestinal Comfort Tea?

If tea is in a bag or a pouch, watch out. Most modern tea bags contain highly processed herbs that are milled down to a powder. Due to the destructive nature of modern processing techniques, this "herbal tea dust" is nearly void of all the medicinal and therapeutic benefits that were once present in the original whole herbs.

Most tea bags are bleached with chlorine to make them white. However, when you steep these bleached tea bags in hot water, toxins like dioxin and epichlorohydrin are released into the water. These chemicals are known to increase risk of many diseases, including cancer.

Study: Plastic tea bags release harmful microplastic particles into hot water

Also, you may have seen a new variety of clear pyramid-shaped "silky tea bags". While these are fancy, more expensive tea bags, that "silky" material is made from plastic.

Researchers from McGill University in Montreal, Canada did a study where they placed the empty tea bags in hot water (95°C or 203°F). They steeped one bag the way you would normally steep your tea. What they found was shocking. A single plastic tea bag released approximately 11.6 billion microplastic particles into the hot water.[2]

The scary thing is that these particles cannot be seen with the naked eye. So, you ingest these microplastics along with your cup of tea. Do you still want to drink from these fancy tea bags? I don't. That is why I drink loose tea exclusively; I just use a steel strainer to remove the herbs after steeping.

"Instant tea powders" are even worse: instant teas are often loaded with chemicals, artificial flavors, & harmful sweeteners to hide poor quality ingredients. Instant tea is also processed using extreme heat, toxic flow agents, and harmful synthetic chemicals to speed up production and cut manufacturing costs.

Therefore, don't waste your time and money on tea bags or "instant tea powders".

I know, for many people it's hard to start drinking loose tea because tea bags and instant tea powders are so convenient and easy to use. But if you are truly on a path to ultimate wellness, straining your loose tea is a small price to pay for being well and feeling good.

How to Take Intestinal Comfort Tea

1. Add 3 leveled tablespoons of Intestinal Comfort Tea to a glass-lined thermos or French press.
2. Add 3 cups of boiling water. Steep the tea for at least 30 minutes.
3. Strain herbs before drinking.
4. Drink 1 cup, 3 times daily: 20 minutes before breakfast, 20 minutes before lunch, and at bedtime.
5. Drink 3 cups of Intestinal Comfort Tea for 21 days. Then, stop for 10 days. Repeat the cycle for the next 12 months.

Immunity G7 Formula™

What is the Immunity G7 Formula?

Immunity G7 Formula is a proprietary blend of pure essential oils, including 100% certified organic European oregano oil, and therapeutic grade true cinnamon oil.

What does Immunity G7 Formula do?

Immunity G7 Formula contains wild oregano oil and cinnamon oil, so it can work as a natural antibiotic/antifungal. Immunity G7 Formula is extremely effective in supporting and boosting the immune system. A strong immune system can protect you from harmful bacteria, viruses, and fungus.

It is encased in easy-to-digest, potent EuroCaps®. This is patented encapsulation technology that allows sealing of oil in a hard gelatin capsule without chemicals, heat, or oxygen. This type of encapsulation ensures that the oil retains freshness and therapeutic potency. Additionally, Immunity G7 Formula has no excipients, solvents, or GMO ingredients.

What is carvacrol in oregano oil, and why does it matter?

Immunity G7 Formula contains organic oregano certified in Europe by EcoCert®. This oil has the highest naturally occurring carvacrol (80+%). Carvacrol is the main chemical compound in wild oregano responsible for inhibiting growth of harmful pathogens (bacteria, fungus). The amount of carvacrol in oregano oil can vary from as little as 10% to as high as 80+%. For oregano oil to work as a therapeutic agent, carvacrol must be above 75%. Most studies use oregano oil with a high concentration of carvacrol.

Study: Oregano Oil as Effective as Traditional Antibiotics against Bacteria

Georgetown University published 2 studies that have shown that oil of oregano "may be an effective treatment against dangerous, and sometimes drug-resistant bacteria", and "carvacrol, one of oregano's chemical components—appear to reduce infection as effectively as traditional antibiotics".[3]

Study: Oregano Oil can be an effective treatment against Candida albica infections.

Candida albicans overgrowth can result in yeast infection in the digestive system, vagina or mouth. It can also cause joint pain, fatigue and mental fog.

In 2001, the Journal of Molecular and Cellular Biochemistry published a study where mice were cured of systemic Candida albicans yeast infection by ingesting oregano oil daily for a month. Furthermore, oregano oil was compared against antifungal antibiotics such as nystatin and amphotericin B. The results were promising. Oregano oil "can act as a potent antifungal agent against C. albicans, and can function similarly to antifungal antibiotics." [4]

Study: Oregano and Thyme Essential Oils Reduce Inflammation in Mice with Colitis

A study published in Mediators of Inflammation in 2007 shows that colitis-afflicted mice experienced less intestinal inflammation, improved integrity of colon tissue, and accelerated weight gain after administration of oregano oil and thyme oil.

So, the results of the study indicated that oral administration of essential oils of oregano and thyme can be useful therapy in inflammatory gut conditions.[5]

Cinnamon is another important ingredient used in Immunity G7 Formula. It has fantastic anti-inflammatory and antimicrobial properties.

Study: Cinnamon Reduces Inflammatory Response in Intestinal Cells.

In IBD, impaired tissue repair and chronic inflammation may result in accumulation of excessive scar tissue within the intestinal wall. This is called intestinal fibrosis.

The only treatment available today for intestinal fibrosis is surgery. Today, no other alternative treatments are available for IBD patients.

German scientists from University of Hohenheim in Stuttgart used cinnamon extract as a therapy for intestinal fibrosis in mice with colitis. They found that "cinnamon decreases fibrotic symptoms", and cinnamon extract "could be potential antifibrotic agents in chronic colitis." [6]

How to Take Immunity G-7 Formula™

1. Start Immunity G7 Formula at the beginning of the Transitional Phase.
2. Take 1 capsule with meals, 3 times daily. If taking 1 capsules 3 times daily are too much for you, reduce the dosage to 1 capsule 1-2 times daily.
3. Do this for 20 days. Then, stop for 10 days. Repeat the cycle for the next 6 months.

Medicinal Clay™

What is Medicinal Clay?

This proprietary formula is a carefully crafted blend of Montmorillonite Sodium & Calcium Bentonite clays from the smectite family. These healing clays come from pristine subterranean deposits (typically 100-1200 feet deep) to ensure purity and optimal health benefits. Medicinal Clay also complies with ANSI/NSF 60 standards for superior quality & safety.

What does Medicinal Clay do?

Medicinal Clay carries a uniquely strong negative ionic charge which causes it to attract any substance with a positive ionic charge (e.g., bacteria, toxins, metals, etc.). These substances are both absorbed (drawn inside), and adsorbed (sticking to the outside like Velcro) by the clay molecules. Your body doesn't digest clay, so the clay passes through your system, collecting toxins, and removing them as the clay is eliminated. Medicinal Clay has a high pH of 8.5-10, which helps shift your body from an acid to an alkaline state.

Clay has been used for centuries as a treatment for diarrhea. During World War II, in the absence of medication, soldiers used clay to successfully fight dysentery. Clay was also used in China as early as the 17th Century as a cure for diarrhea.

Medicinal Clay can work wonders for ulcerative colitis and Crohn's disease patients.

Taken internally as a drink, Medicinal Clay works like a sponge by soaking up parasites, bacteria, mold, and the buildup of toxic waste, all of which are then excreted from your body in your poop. This deep cleansing and detoxification optimize the body's natural healing abilities, improves organ function, optimizes tissue repair, reduces harmful acids, and boosts energy. As a result, you'll find that diarrhea, abdominal cramps, nausea, and overall fatigue are greatly reduced.

Study: "The Value of Bentonite for Diarrhea"

In this study, clay proved to be effective in halting diarrhea in 97% of patients in about 4 days. Sixty years ago, Dr. Damrau of New York City published a study called "The Value of Bentonite for Diarrhea". In this study, the therapeutic effect of bentonite for acute diarrhea was evaluated in 35 patients afflicted with virus infections, food allergy, food poisoning, spastic or mucous colitis. Patients took 2 Tablespoons of bentonite, mixed with distilled water, 3 times daily. "Acute diarrhea was relieved in 34 out of 35 cases (97%) on an average period of 3.8 days, ranging from 1-4 days. No side-effects to bentonite drinks were observed in any of the patients."

That's truly amazing![7]

How to Prepare Medicinal Clay drink for Diarrhea:

The Medicinal Clay drink will help stop your diarrhea and cleanse your body from toxins. Drink daily for 14 days or until your diarrhea is resolved.

Ingredients/Supplies:

- 1 glass jar (at least quart-sized)
- 3 heaping Tablespoons of Medicinal Clay
- Non-metal Tablespoon (wooden, ceramic, or plastic)
- 1 liter or 32 ounces (4 cups) of boiled filtered or boiled spring water

Directions:

1. Add 1 liter boiled, cooled water to a glass jar.
2. Using the non-metal tablespoon, add 3 heaping tablespoons of Medicinal Clay to the water. (Do not use metal containers or utensils; contact with metal decreases the clay's potency.)
3. Mix the Medicinal Clay with the boiled water very well, and let it sit for 6-8 hours or overnight on the counter. This allows the Medicinal Clay to diffuse and charge the water.
4. Before drinking, stir well.
5. Drink 3 cups daily: 1 cup first thing in the morning on an empty stomach, 1 cup between meals, and 1 cup at bedtime.
6. Repeat daily for 14 days or until your diarrhea is resolved.

Colon Formula™

What is the Colon Formula?

This 100% organic, extra-strength formula was designed to support healthy intestinal flora and to protect against parasites and harmful bacteria. It is a specially sourced and processed combination of organic cloves and organic wormwood. It is gluten-free, non-GMO, kosher, with no heavy metals, and no excipients.

The benefits of Colon Cleansing Drink

- Stops diarrhea, abdominal cramps and bloating
- Defends against parasites and harmful bacteria
- Supports healthy intestinal flora

Study: Taking wormwood supplement results in complete remission in 65% of Crohn's disease patients.

Wormwood was used in a German double-blind study on 40 patients with Crohn's disease. These patients were taking steroids daily. The patients were divided into 2 treatment groups. For 10 weeks, one group received an herbal blend containing wormwood at a dose of 500 milligrams, 3 times per day, plus steroids. The second group received a placebo, plus steroids.

What researchers found was shocking: after 8 weeks of treatment, 90% of the patients who took wormwood experienced steady improvement and 65% had almost complete remission of symptoms. Patients taking wormwood were able to decrease or even eliminate the need for steroids. Moreover, patients who took wormwood experienced improved mood and quality of life, which cannot be done with steroids.

On the other hand, the condition of patients who received a placebo got worse after the tapering of steroids, and 80% of patients in the placebo group were forced to restart steroids after week 10.[8]

How to Take Colon Formula

1. Before taking, cover each capsule with a little butter or coconut oil - the fat will allow for better absorption.
2. Take 2 capsules, 3 times daily, with chicken broth or soup. Do this for 14 days or until your diarrhea is resolved. If taking 2 capsules 3 times daily are too much for you, reduce the dosage to 1 capsule 3 times daily.

Arctic Cod Liver Oil

What is Arctic Cod Liver Oil?

Nordic Naturals Arctic Cod Liver Oil is fish oil from Norway that is molecularly distilled and enhanced with antioxidants for freshness and great taste. This product has the highest level of Omega-3 fatty acids per teaspoon of any cod liver oil, with only naturally occurring vitamins A and D. Nordic Naturals products surpass all national and international pharmaceutical standards for freshness and purity, and are free from heavy metals, dioxins, and PCBs. Carlson Cod Liver Oil is another brand you can buy if you cannot find Nordic Naturals Arctic Cod Liver Oil.

Studies show that fish oil has strong anti-inflammatory action in IBD

Studies show marked improvement in active ulcerative colitis after fish oil supplementation. Ulcerative colitis is accompanied by an increased level of leukotriene B4 in the lining of the colon. Fish oils are known to inhibit the synthesis of leukotrienes, and so, they might be beneficial in the treatment of ulcerative colitis.

Researchers at the Veterans Affairs Medical Center released the results of a study aimed at testing this hypothesis. The study involved 11 male patients aged 31 to 74 years old, who had been diagnosed with ulcerative colitis. The patients were randomized into two groups, with one group receiving 15 fish oil capsules providing 2.7 grams of eicosatetraenoic acid (EPA) and 1.8 grams of docosahexaenoic acid (DHA) daily. The other group received placebo capsules (olive oil). After 3 months on the supplements, all participants underwent a 2-month wash-out period and were then assigned the opposite treatment they had received during the first stage for another 3 months.

Clinical evaluations of all patients were performed at the start of the study and every month thereafter. Evaluation of the patients' clinical data at the end of the treatment periods showed a significant beneficial effect of fish oil supplementation. The mean disease severity score for patients on fish oil declined by 56%, as compared to 4% for the placebo group.

8 of the 11 patients (72%) were able to markedly reduce or eliminate their use of anti-inflammatory medication and steroids while taking the fish oils.

The researchers concluded that fish oil supplementation results in a marked clinical improvement of active mild to moderate ulcerative colitis.[9]

How to Take Arctic Cod Liver Oil

1. Take 1 teaspoon of fish oil with fresh vegetable juice, 2-3 times a day. Please don't use factory-made bottled juice.
2. For maintenance, once diarrhea has ceased, you can increase your dosage of cod liver oil to 1 tablespoon a day. It can be taken with fresh vegetable juice.

Activated Charcoal

What is Activated Charcoal and what are its benefits?

Activated charcoal is a fine odorless black powder made from burning carbon-based materials such as coconut shells or wood at high temperature with the addition of calcium chloride.

Activated charcoal works through the process of adsorption, which is the reaction that promotes binding of different substances to the surface of the charcoal. Bacteria, toxins, and intestinal gas have a positive electric charge, whereas activated charcoal has a negative charge. As you know, opposite charges attract. So, the porous surface of activated charcoal literally traps bacteria, toxins, and gas, and safely eliminates them from the digestive system with a stool. Activated Charcoal works so well as a binding agent that hospitals even use it on patients who are suffering from drug overdoses. It works exceptionally well for the following:

- Elimination of excessive gas, bloating and diarrhea
- Removal of toxins (pesticides and fungicides sprayed on food)
- Removal of chemicals (from water, food, and the environment)
- Detoxification and cleansing of the gastrointestinal system and kidneys

European Food Safety Authority (EFSA) Report

Based on 3 human intervention studies, a report concluded that activated charcoal can be used for reduction of excessive intestinal gas and bloating in the general population. Also, charcoal is "traditionally used to contribute to good digestive comfort."[10]

The EFSA recommends taking 1 gram of activated charcoal before and after a meal.

I use the dosage of activated charcoal recommended by the EFSA during The Flare Stopper System.

Study: Activated Charcoal for Diarrhea

Activated charcoal is an effective and suitable treatment for diarrhea, according to a 2017 review of recent studies found on PubMed and MEDLINE. Diarrhea can be caused by irritable bowel syndrome, bacterial infection, and chemotherapy.

Activated charcoal can absorb and clear bacteria and various toxins that cause diarrhea. Furthermore, "In comparison, with other common anti-diarrheal treatments, activated charcoal has exceptionally few side-effects." This makes activated charcoal a safe and effective treatment for diarrhea.[11]

How to use Activated Charcoal

1. Take 2 capsules (500mg each) 1 hour before meals with 8oz water. Do 3 times daily for 5 days during Introduction Phase. (You should take a total of 6 capsules a day.)
2. Drink at least 8-10 cups of water a day with 1 tablespoon of fresh lemon juice in each cup, to ensure that toxins and chemicals are flushed from your body.
3. Please note: charcoal can turn your stool black.

Colon Cleansing Drink

What is Colon Cleansing Drink?

Colon Cleansing Drink has 2 ingredients: powdered psyllium husk and liquid bentonite.

The benefits of Colon Cleansing Drink

- Reduces intestinal inflammation bloating, and loose stools
- Supports healthy intestinal flora
- Prolongs IBD remissions

Liquid Bentonite

Liquid bentonite has powerful adsorption (physical binding) properties. Because bentonite retains its negative charge, it can effectively bind positively charged substances such as metabolic, environmental, and chemical toxins from the digestive tract. You can use bentonite made by the Yerba Prima company or Sonne's #7 Bentonite.

Psyllium Husk

Psyllium husk is the outer layer of the psyllium seed, and it's made by milling the seed to remove the husk. Psyllium husk is a bulk-forming fiber that promotes healthy and easy stool elimination. It contains mostly soluble fiber that can be used daily to give bulk to your stool and to promote normal stool elimination. Because it has no laxative stimulants, it does not overstimulate the peristaltic muscles of the bowel, and it does not create "dependency" as herbal laxatives do.

Psyllium husk works like a sponge by gently absorbing buildup of toxins from your colon walls. It eliminates both constipation and diarrhea. Psyllium can soften hardened stool attached to the mucous lining of the bowel wall, which can help with constipation and stool elimination. Your stool should be of a perfect consistency - not too loose, not too firm, and should look like a thick sausage.

Adding psyllium to your diet may reduce the risk of heart disease and lower the risk of colon cancer. It can be used daily.

Psyllium husk has similar properties to the Psyllium seed used in the study below. Instead of psyllium husk, you can also use organic, powdered psyllium seed powder sold online or in health food stores.

Study: Psyllium Seed is Effective in Maintaining UC Remission

According to a Spanish study, published in the American Journal of Gastroenterology, psyllium seed supplementation given to people with ulcerative colitis was as effective in maintaining remission as anti-inflammatory medication (mesalamine). It was found that taking psyllium seed supplementation (10 grams twice daily) increased levels of butyric acid.[12]

How to Make Intestinal Cleansing Drink

Ingredients/Supplies:

- 1 heaping teaspoon of psyllium husk powder
- 16 ounces of warm boiled water (to be used for 2 separate drinks)
- 1 Tablespoon of liquid bentonite

Directions:

1. In 8 ounces of warm boiled water, add 1 heaping teaspoon of psyllium powder. Stir briskly and drink immediately.
2. In another 8 ounces of warm boiled water, add 1 Tablespoon of bentonite. Stir well, and drink right away.
3. Drink this duo (the first cup with psyllium, the second cup with bentonite) twice daily: first thing in the morning and at night before bedtime.

Conclusion

Now you've learned about using supplements as tools to repair the damaged gastrointestinal mucosa, lower overall level of inflammation, and restore digestive health.

Next, we will learn about therapies.

References

[1] Chakŭrski, I et al. "Lechenie na bolni s khronichni koliti s bilkova kombinatsiia ot Taraxacum officinale, Hipericum perforatum, Melissa officinalis, Calendula officinalis, Foeniculum vulgare" [Treatment of chronic colitis with an herbal combination of Taraxacum officinale, Hipericum perforatum, Melissa officinaliss, Calendula officinalis and Foeniculum vulgare]. *Vutreshni bolesti* vol. 20,6 (1981): 51-4.
https://www.ncbi.nlm.nih.gov/pubmed/7336706

[2] Hernandez, Laura M et al. "Plastic Teabags Release Billions of Microparticles and Nanoparticles into Tea." *Environmental science & technology* vol. 53,21 (2019): 12300-12310. doi:10.1021/acs.est.9b02540

[3] Georgetown University Medical Center. "Oregano Oil May Protect Against Drug-Resistant Bacteria, Georgetown Researcher Finds." *ScienceDaily*. ScienceDaily, 11 October 2001. www.sciencedaily.com/releases/2001/10/011011065609.htm

[4] Manohar, V et al. "Antifungal activities of origanum oil against Candida albicans." *Molecular and cellular biochemistry* vol. 228,1-2 (2001): 111-7. doi:10.1023/a:1013311632207

[5] Bukovská, Alexandra et al. "Effects of a combination of thyme and oregano essential oils on TNBS-induced colitis in mice." *Mediators of inflammation* vol. 2007 (2007): 23296. doi:10.1155/2007/23296

[6] Hagenlocher, Yvonne et al. "Cinnamon reduces inflammatory response in intestinal fibroblasts in vitro and in colitis in vivo leading to decreased fibrosis." *Molecular nutrition & food research* vol. 61,9 (2017): 10.1002/mnfr.201601085. doi:10.1002/mnfr.201601085
https://pubmed.ncbi.nlm.nih.gov/28324642/

[7] Frederic Damrau M.D., "The Value of Bentonite for Diarrhea." *Medical Annals of The District of Columbia* Vol. 30, No. 6, June, 1961

[8] Omer, B et al. "Steroid-sparing effect of wormwood (Artemisia absinthium) in Crohn's disease: a double-blind placebo-controlled study." *Phytomedicine: international journal of phytotherapy and phytopharmacology* vol. 14,2-3 (2007): 87-95. doi:10.1016/j.phymed.2007.01.001
https://www.ncbi.nlm.nih.gov/pubmed/17240130

[9] Aslan, A, and G Triadafilopoulos. "Fish oil fatty acid supplementation in active ulcerative colitis: a double-blind, placebo-controlled, crossover study." *The American journal of gastroenterology* vol. 87,4 (1992): 432-7.

[10] https://efsa.onlinelibrary.wiley.com/doi/pdf/10.2903/j.efsa.2011.2049

[11] Senderovich, Helen, and Megan J Vierhout. "Is there a role for charcoal in palliative diarrhea management?." *Current medical research and opinion* vol. 34,7 (2018): 1253-1259. doi:10.1080/03007995.2017.1416345
https://pubmed.ncbi.nlm.nih.gov/29231746/

[12] Fernández-Bañares F, et al. "Randomized clinical trial of Plantago ovata seeds (dietary fiber) as compared with mesalamine in maintaining remission in ulcerative colitis." Spanish Group for the Study of Crohn's Disease and Ulcerative Colitis (GETECCU). *Am J Gastroenterol.* 1999 Feb;94(2):427-33. doi: 10.1111/j.1572-0241.1999.872_a.x. PMID: 10022641.
https://www.ncbi.nlm.nih.gov/pubmed/10022641

CHAPTER 12

Therapies

IN ADDITION TO DIET AND SUPPLEMENTS, YOU WILL ALSO BE DOING various therapies to promote intestinal healing and normalization of bowel movements. These therapies include the following:

- Medicinal Clay Abdominal Application (Poultice)
- Ileocecal Valve (ICV) Adjustment
- Therapeutic Enemas for IBD
- Ozone Therapy in IBD

Please read below why these therapies are important.

Medicinal Clay™ Abdominal Application (Poultice)

The Medicinal Clay™ poultice is an application of clay paste on a person's abdomen, which is kept in place for 2 hours. You create this paste by mixing Medicinal Clay with water. This poultice is used to draw out toxins and reduce overall inflammation. During a flare, it must be done daily for at least 21 days. I find it relaxing to do the clay poultice application in the evening.

You'll find directions below on how to make the Medicinal Clay poultice. You can also follow along with an instructional video I've added to my website: knowyourgut.com/video/.

How to Prepare Medicinal Clay Poultice for Abdominal Application

Here is the list of ingredients and supplies that you need for Medicinal Clay poultice.

Ingredients/Supplies:

- Non-metal Tablespoon (wooden, ceramic, or plastic)
- Non-metal bowl (glass, ceramic, or plastic)
- 7-10 heaping Tablespoons of Medicinal Clay
- 7-10 Tablespoons of filtered water (cooled after boiling)
- Clean white cotton cloth
- Clear plastic wrap
- Self-adherent elastic wrap/bandage

Directions:

1. Using a non-metal spoon, measure 7-10 heaping tablespoons of clay into a non-metal bowl. (Do not use metal containers or utensils; contact with metal decreases the clay's potency.) Add about 10 Tablespoons of warm filtered water to the bowl. Mix well with the Medicinal Clay. The clay mixture should be smooth, the consistency of thick sour cream without lumps. Add more water if needed.
2. Apply ½ inch thick of clay mixture to your abdomen.
3. Cover the clay mixture that is spread on your abdomen with a clean, cotton cloth. Then, cover that cloth with a big piece of

clear plastic wrap. Then, wrap an elastic bandage around your entire midsection to hold everything in place.

4. Lay down with this Medicinal Clay poultice for about 2 hours.
5. After 2 hours, carefully unwind the bandage and remove the poultice. You can scoop off the clay from your abdomen, and discard. Rinse off the remaining clay using warm water. You might have slight redness on your skin, which will go away soon.

Ileocecal Valve (ICV) Adjustment

What is the ileocecal valve (ICV)?

The ileocecal valve (ICV) is a sphincter muscle that connects the small intestine to the large intestine. It works like a gate that opens when digested food from the small intestine is ready to move into the large intestine. After the digested food is passed, the ICV closes. For a healthy person, the ICV is a one-way street.

A healthy ileocecal valve stops food in the large intestine from backing up to the small intestine. Since the food material in the large intestine contains waste and toxins, it should stay in the large intestine until it's excreted with stool. In people with ulcerative colitis and Crohn's disease, the ileocecal valve usually malfunctions. It becomes inflamed and stays open.

And a terrible thing happens!

The waste material from the large intestine backs up into the small intestine. After this happens, food (together with toxins from the large intestine) starts rotting in the small intestine, causing small intestinal bacterial overgrowth (SIBO), bloating, abdominal pain, and malabsorption of nutrients. Furthermore, toxins get absorbed from the walls of the small intestine, directly into your bloodstream, causing liver dysfunction. This causes even more digestive problems, such as heartburn, acid reflux, and burping.

Even in the absence of flares, I suffered from ICV inflammation and malfunction for years, and did not know it. I took good quality supplements, ate a healthy diet, and still - I suffered from malabsorption, gas, bloating, abdominal pain, and right shoulder pain. I could not understand what was wrong with me. It was only years later that I discovered my inflamed ICV was the reason why I felt so lousy.

In order to restore the health of your digestive system, the function of your ICV must be fully restored.

Where is the ileocecal valve located?

Draw a straight line between your right hip bone and your belly button. Your ICV is located in the middle of that line, in the lower right side of your abdomen.

What are the causes of ileocecal valve inflammation?

ICV inflammation can be caused by:

- Eating junk food
- Spine misalignment
- Food allergies & intolerances
- Parasitic and bacterial infections
- Emotional & psychological stress
- Drinking too many caffeinated beverages
- Overeating and/or eating too fast without proper chewing

An inflamed ICV is the hidden cause of many health problems

Special attention should be given to correction of ileocecal valve (ICV) malfunction. There is a close relationship between a healthy gut and a properly aligned spine and muscles. An open and inflamed ileocecal valve is one of the root causes of ongoing dysbiosis, diarrhea, and bloating in IBD patients.

This condition is also known to cause persistent Candida albicans problems, joint pain similar to arthritis, chronic fatigue, migraine headaches, and right shoulder pain. Unfortunately, ICV inflammation is often overlooked by doctors. They rarely correlate ICV problems with ongoing numerous health problems. So, it's up to you to find a good chiropractor qualified in proper ICV adjustment.

How can you restore the healthy function of the ileocecal valve?

The best time to address the inflammation of your ICV is while you are doing this program. You can address ICV malfunction by doing two things simultaneously:

- Reduce inflammation of the entire gastrointestinal system by following instructions in this book (The Flare Stopper System).
- Undergo ICV adjustments by a chiropractor, thereby retraining your ICV to function properly. A knowledgeable chiropractor will be able to restore ICV function by doing adjustments to affected areas of your abdomen and spine. In cases of open valve problems, I find it helpful to place a cold pack over the valve for 5-10 minutes prior to chiropractic adjustment.

ICV Self-massage

In the absence of a qualified chiropractor, you can do ICV self-massage.

Directions:

1. Locate your ICV with your fingers - it's at the midpoint between your right hip bone and your belly button.

2. Place a cold pack over the ICV for about 5-10 minutes prior to your adjustment. After you've finished with the cold pack, put it aside.
3. Lie on your back with your knees bent.
4. Locate your ICV again. Using 3 fingers, press into the ICV. If it's inflamed, this area will be swollen and painful.
5. Press deep into your skin into the ICV area, and pull strongly, diagonally toward the belly button. Hold for 1 minute.
6. Repeat a few more times.
7. Then, massage over the ICV area in a clockwise direction until the ICV area stops being tender to touch.

Therapeutic Enemas for IBD

To comply with the current position of conventional GI doctors, at the time of the flare in ulcerative colitis and Crohn's disease, I recommend small, therapeutic retention enemas. Enemas can help you disinfect your colon and lower GI inflammation by physically moving toxins and pathogens out of the body quickly.

When done correctly, enema promotes healthy gut flora, optimizes the microbiome, and has a cleansing, detoxifying effect on the whole body.

What are Enemas?

When I tell my patients that they must do enemas, most of them ask, "What is it?" and "Why should we do it?".

An enema is a method of introducing liquid into the rectum to physically remove pathogenic organisms and old, impacted toxic waste buildup lodged in the folds of the intestines.

Why does toxic waste buildup happen?

Our gastrointestinal system is constantly under stress due to poor nutrition, low fiber diets, inadequate chewing, processed foods, GMO foods, chemical additives, and preservatives. Junk food affects the health of intestinal lining, and with time, the intestinal wall gets covered with hardened waste that blocks absorption of nutrients.

Why should you do Enemas?

The truth is, in IBD the colon is in a state of dysbiosis (altered gut flora). As we have discussed before, the presence of pathogens (harmful bacteria, fungi, viruses, and parasites) is common in people with Crohn's disease and colitis. Intestinal inflammation is exacerbated by the continuous presence of these pathogens.

An enema cleanses and detoxifies the colon, thereby reducing disease-causing pathogens in the gut. It is impossible to heal an inflamed colon entirely without getting rid of the epicenters of infection and toxicity caused by pathogens. To allow your intestinal wall to heal, first you absolutely MUST remove pathogens that live, eat, and poop in your gut.

Because intestinal cells are renewed every 4-5 days, you can speed up the gut healing process by using enemas to allow for direct contact of gut-healing herbs with your colon lining. People usually start feeling better quickly once the pathogenic flora and toxic waste materials are removed from their colon.

Doctors approve Therapeutic Retention Enemas & Colon Cleansing

Naturopathic Doctor, Mark Davis states:

> *"Two-thirds of UC patients have distal disease, confined to the left side of the colon. Therapeutic retention enemas*

are highly indicated for this population, but may also be utilized for patients with more extensive disease, up to and including pancolitis. Rectally-administered therapies are underutilized in IBD, due in part to physician perception of patient unwillingness to use them, and embarrassment in discussing rectal modalities; however, in my practice I've prescribed and administered hundreds of enemas and found them to be extremely helpful in the treatment of UC, especially left-sided UC and ulcerative proctitis, the latter of which is notoriously stubborn to medical management." [1]

Gastrointestinal surgeon, Dr. Leonard Smith on colon hydrotherapy:

Dr. Leonard Smith has extensive experience in operating on patients with different GI pathologies, including colon cancer, diverticulitis, appendicitis, hemorrhoids, and other GI problems. Here is his opinion on colon hydrotherapy:

> *"Without any reservation, I declare that my wish is to see colon hydrotherapy as an established procedure for many kinds of gastrointestinal problems. If medical centers, hospitals, and clinics installed colon hydrotherapy departments, they would find such departments just as efficacious for patients as their present treatment areas which are devoted to physiotherapy. Such is my true belief, and I do endorse this therapeutic program."* [2]

Naturopathic Doctor, Pamela Whitney, recommends Colon Cleansing

Pamela Whitney, ND is educational director for the New England Health Institute. She is a naturopathic physician who practices in Braintree, Massachusetts.

Dr. Whitney says:

> *"Most people possess toxic bowels which may result in either constipation or diarrhea both coming from the same sources of toxicity."*

Dr. Whitney describes how it works: "Using hydrotherapy, the colon's walls constantly get flushed with clear fluid, which serves to remove mucus plus some of their longstanding, caked-on fecal matter which contains hidden bacteria, parasites, Candida albicans-filled pockets, and other such pathological materials" [2]

What are the Benefits of Enemas/ Colon Hydrotherapy?

- Elimination of toxins and lowering microbial load
- Relief of gas, bloating, diarrhea and abdominal pain
- Normalization and rebalancing of intestinal microflora

In this program, we use 2 types of enemas

1. Cleansing enema
2. Medicinal retention enema

The Purpose of Cleansing Enema with Salt

This enema's purpose is to gently flush stool, toxins and pathogenic intestinal microflora from the colon.

The Purpose of Therapeutic Retention Enema with Colon Formula™

This enema is used to deliver medicinal herbs directly to the colon, so it can be directly absorbed by the mucous lining of the intestines. The herbs used in this enema are very potent. Studies show that Colon

Formula™ herbs have antimicrobial, antifungal, antiparasitic and anti-inflammatory effects.[3, 4]

When to Administer Cleansing and Retention Enemas

Both enemas are administered once a day - in the morning right after your first bowel movement. If you have multiple bowel movements in the morning, then wait until you have no urges to run to the bathroom. If your rectum is sore, rest for 1-2 hours before you start administering enemas. The duration of this daily enema program is from 7 to 30 days, depending on the condition of the patient. In this program, the cleansing enemas are used for 21 days in a row.

Important: First, you clear your bowels using cleansing enema. Then, you follow-up with a therapeutic retention enema to disinfect the intestinal wall and to soothe the inflamed, ulcerated colon. Do not use tap water, because it may contain chemicals that are harmful for your colon.

Supplies you will need to do 2 enemas

- Two Disposable Enema bottles, about 4.5 oz (Fleet is a common brand sold in any pharmacy)
- 2 enamel pots with lids
- 2 cups of filtered or store-bought spring water
- ¼ teaspoon of Himalayan salt
- 2 capsules of Colon Formula™
- Yoga mat
- Towels*
- Small pillow (optional)
- Heater (optional)
- Relaxing music and candles (optional)

Note: I prefer to use white towels - it's easier to wash them later with laundry detergent and bleach.

How to Set up for an Enema

The best place to do an enema is in your bathroom, since the urge to poop may come on rather quickly.

1. On the floor of the bathroom, lay down a yoga mat.
2. Place 2 towels on the mat, and a small pillow, so you'll be comfortable while doing the enema.
3. If it's cold in your bathroom, turn on a small heater, so the temperature inside the bathroom is warm. For a more pleasant experience, you can turn on relaxing music and light up some candles.

How to Prepare a Cleansing Enema

1. In an enamel pot, boil 1 cup (8 ounces) of water for 5 minutes.
2. Add 1/4 teaspoon of Himalayan salt to 1 cup of hot water.
3. Stir well with dry, clean poon to ensure that all the salt is dissolved fully.
4. Let it cool to room temperature before using it for enema. The water should be 25-30 degrees Celsius or 77-86 Fahrenheit. If it's too cold or too hot, it will cause a spasm in your intestines.
5. Prepare a disposable Fleet enema bottle. Each bottle holds about 4.5 ounces. Unscrew the top of an enema; discard the liquid content of the bottle.
6. Then, using a clean, dry funnel, pour 4 oz of salty, cooled water into one empty enema bottle, and screw the top back on.
7. Now, you are ready to administer your cleansing enema.

How to Prepare Therapeutic Retention Enema

1. In an enamel pot, boil 1 cup (8 ounces) of water.
2. Wash your hands with hot water and soap. Dry your hand with paper towels.
3. Open 2 capsules of Colon Formula™ and add herbs from the capsules into the boiling water. Discard the empty capsules. Mix well with a clean spoon.

4. Turn the heat off and cover the pot with a lid; let stand for 1 hour on the counter.
5. Then, strain out the herbs into a dry, clean, glass measuring cup with spout.
6. Prepare a disposable Fleet enema bottle. Each bottle holds about 4.5 oz.
7. Unscrew the top of an enema; discard the liquid content of the bottle.
8. Then, using a clean, dry funnel, pour 4 oz of the herbal liquid from a glass measuring cup into one empty enema bottle, and screw the top back on.
9. Make sure the liquid inside the enema is room temperature. Do not use it if it's warm. Otherwise, you'll be running to the bathroom.

How to Administer a Cleansing Enema and Therapeutic Retention Enema

1. Prepare your enema solution.
2. Lie on your left side, with your left leg bent. Slowly, gently, insert the lubricated enema tip into your rectum. Do not force it. Squeeze the bottle until it is empty. Relax and breathe deeply. Let the mixture flow freely into your bowels.
3. Remove enema tip gently, and try to retain the enema while you are lying in the left-sided position for 2-3 minutes.
4. If you feel you need to expel some stool, quickly get up and sit on the toilet. You might see rubber-like pieces of stool, small chunks of stool, some blood, and lots of mucus.
5. After the cleansing enema is completed, you can rest for 5-10 minutes.
6. Then, follow-up with administration of a Therapeutic Retention Enema containing Colon Formula™ herbal solution. Follow the procedure described above. Try to retain Therapeutic Retention Enema for 15-20 minutes.
7. Administer both cleansing enemas and therapeutic enemas daily for 21 days.

What to Expect after Administration of Enemas?

You must understand that the tissues of your bowel are saturated with mucus and toxins that have been stored there for years of your sickness. Whenever this mucus is released, you will usually see some bleeding associated with mucus being purged from the walls of your intestines. That happens because, with the release of deeper layers of mucus, the colon ulcers are being exposed, ready to be healed. However, bleeding can increase from these exposed ulcers. That's why therapeutic retention enema is necessary to disinfect and heal the mucous lining of the colon.

Conclusion

Enemas, when used daily for 21 days, may contribute to remission in ulcerative colitis and Crohn's disease. People with mild or moderate disease activity may be most likely to observe the quick improvement of the symptoms such as decreased bleeding, abdominal spasms and BM's urgency.

Ozone Therapy for IBD

If you have the means, you can add ozone therapy during a transitional stage of the program to accelerate your healing. It's not a prerequisite but it's a very powerful, supportive solution.

What is Ozone Therapy?

Ozone is a colorless gas that is composed of three oxygen atoms. Regular oxygen is made up of two oxygen atoms. It is the third oxygen atom that makes ozone "supercharged" oxygen, and gives it all of its phenomenal medical properties.

Ozone therapy has been used in medicine for over 125 years to treat wounds, infections, autoimmune diseases, and other chronic health problems.

What most people don't know is that ozone works by increasing oxygen utilization in your body. This helps purify the blood and lymph fluids, improve circulation, reduce pain, improve digestion, elimination, and production of hormones and enzymes.

The use of ozone in medicine is based on the fact that toxins are removed by the process of oxidation.

Here is what happens in your body: oxidation breaks toxins down into carbon dioxide and water, which are eliminated from your body. However, if you are chronically sick, your body is usually deficient in oxygen. Therefore, you cannot eliminate toxins adequately, and a toxic buildup occurs. This leads to weakness, fatigue, and a wide range of degenerative diseases.

Problem of Low Oxygen in IBD

In IBD, the intestinal mucosa (lining) undergoes active inflammation; "nutrients and local oxygen become rapidly depleted, resulting in hypoxia" (low oxygen).[5]

That means if you have active IBD inflammation, your intestinal cells increase their consumption of oxygen. This creates the state of hypoxia or oxygen deprivation in the body, which is one of the main reasons why IBD patients often experience weakness, fatigue and low energy. If we want to reverse the disease process in IBD, we must increase oxygen level in the cells. After the body receives enough oxygen, blood flow improves, pathogens (fungus, viruses, bacteria, parasites) die, and the immune system gets restored to its healthy function.

Ozone was used to treat IBD patients back in the 1930's

The use of ozone therapy for IBD is not a new idea or a novel treatment.

"Ozone was the focus of considerable research in Germany during the 1930's where it was successfully used to treat patients suffering from inflammatory bowel disorders, ulcerative colitis, Crohn's disease and chronic bacterial diarrhea." [6]

These doctors were using ozone to treat Crohn's disease, ulcerative colitis, fistula, hemorrhoids, proctitis, and chronic bacterial diarrhea. It was reported that daily introduction of rectal ozone insufflation in the bowel of IBD patients promoted healing of the intestinal lining and restored the balance of intestinal flora.

Millions of ozone treatments have been done in Europe

> *"It is estimated that over 10 million ozone treatments have been given to over 1 million patients in Germany alone over the last 40 years. Today, an estimated 9,000 licensed health practitioners in Germany use ozone. [...] Another 8,000 practitioners across Europe are using it. It is generally given by rectal insufflation, injection, autohemotherapy (in which blood is extracted, treated and then returned to the body), by steam cabinet, body bag and, under special conditions, inhalation."* [7]

Germany, Russia, and Cuba conduct extensive research studies on bio-oxidative therapies. In Europe, ozone therapy has become a part of mainstream medicine in the treatment of many diseases such as atherosclerosis, hypertensive disease, diabetes mellitus, chronic bronchitis, bronchial asthma, chronic gastritis, peptic ulcer, ulcer of the stomach, and chronic colitis.

Benefits of Ozone Therapy for IBD

Studies show the following benefits of ozone on the human body:

1. **Ozone has an anti-inflammatory effect**: it oxidizes the biologically active compounds (arachidonic acid and its derivative, prostaglandins) that participate in the development and sustainment of the inflammatory process.
2. **Ozone is very effective in killing pathogens** such as harmful bacteria, viruses, parasites, and fungus. Ozone kills bacteria by damaging its cell membrane.
3. **Ozone works as a powerful detoxifier**; it activates metabolic processes in the liver and kidneys, which aid these organs of detoxification in removing toxic compounds from the body.
4. **Ozone supports your own immune system** by activating phagocytosis – the process by which the immune system cells engulf pathogens. Ozone also enhances synthesis of the protein interferon, which protects us from viral infections by "interfering" with viral replication.
5. **Ozone improves oxygenation of the tissues.** Ozone increases oxygen saturation of the body's cells. More oxygen inside cells equals more energy in the body.[8]

Therapeutic Applications of Ozone for IBD

The following are simple, inexpensive, and non-invasive ozone treatments for IBD:

- Rectal insufflations with ozone/oxygen mixture
- Drinking of ozonated water

Rectal insufflation with ozone

In 2008, Ministry of Health Service of the Russian Federation published a Health Manual called "Ozone Therapy in Practice". Here is their opinion on rectal ozone therapy:

> *"The use of rectal insufflations with ozone produces both anti-inflammatory and immune balancing effect due to ozone capacity to increase oxygen saturation of the intestinal cells. When rectal insufflations are used ozone gets stuck to the mucous membrane and interferes with the infectious process penetrating the microbial cells thus preventing their further reproduction. Intestinal insufflations can be administered, first of all, as anti-inflammatory and disinfectant remedy to restore the bacterial flora misbalanced by pathogenic microorganisms."*[8]

According to the German Medical Association of Ozone Application, rectal ozone insufflation is "one of the oldest forms of application in ozone therapy. It's recommended to do ozone rectal insufflation for ulcerous colitis, proctitis, anal fistulae and fissures. [9]

Drinking of ozonated water

Ozone has been used to disinfect water since the late 1800s in Europe. According to the Water Research Center:

"Ozone has a greater disinfection effectiveness against bacteria and viruses compared to chlorination."[10]

Fortunately, water treatment with ozone does not add chemicals to the water. Ozonating water allows you to enjoy the benefits of ozone. You can use an ozone water bubbler for ozonating water without allowing ozone to escape into the air. A filter system known as the Ozone Destruct System is also used because excess ozone gas needs to be neutralized in order to reduce irritation.

When ozonating water, it's recommended to use cold distilled water. Cold water will hold ozone for longer periods of time. To receive the maximum effect, it's recommended to drink ozonated water as soon as possible after ozonating. Leftover water should be kept refrigerated.

It will hold the ozone for up to 24 hours; however, it's best to drink ozonated water within the first 1-2 hours.

Where to buy ozone therapy equipment

You can buy the Ozone Therapies Standard Package here:

knowyourgut.com/products/ozone-therapies-standard-package/.

You will also need to buy an oxygen tank to operate the ozone generator. Most people use industrial oxygen, which is 99.2% pure oxygen. Medical oxygen is 99.5% pure oxygen, and it requires a prescription. You can buy an oxygen tank at a local Praxair store, Airgas store, or at a welding supplies store.

Contraindications to ozone therapy

1. All cases with Blood Coagulation Failure (acute and chronic tendency for bleeding)
2. Hemorrhagic or Apoplectic Stroke
3. Ozone Intolerance and/or Allergy
4. Thrombocytopenia
5. Bleeding Organs
6. Hyperthyroidism
7. Leukemia
8. Favism

Important Note: Make sure you do not inhale ozone - if ozone gas goes into your eyes or nose, you can experience coughing, headaches, nausea, vomiting, and a burning sensation in your eyes.

Conclusion

All the therapies written about in this chapter are powerful tools when used as a part of The Flare Stopper System. When used correctly, these therapies can help you reverse the IBD disease process quickly and effectively.

References

[1] Mark Davis, ND, "Therapeutic retention enemas: an underutilized modality for UC". *Naturopathic Doctors News & Review*. Posted 1.11.2016 http://ndnr.com/gastrointestinal/therapeutic-retention-enemas-an-underutilized-modality-for-uc/

[2] Dr. Walker, M. (2000). Value of Colon Hydrotherapy Verified by Medical Professionals. *Townsend Letter for Doctors and Patients*, Aug/Sept Edition

[3] Han, Xuesheng, and Tory L Parker. "Anti-inflammatory activity of clove (Eugenia caryophyllata) essential oil in human dermal fibroblasts." *Pharmaceutical biology* vol. 55,1 (2017): 1619-1622. doi:10.1080/13880209.2017.1314513

[4] Munyangi, Jérôme et al. "Effect of Artemisia annua and Artemisia afra tea infusions on schistosomiasis in a large clinical trial." *Phytomedicine: international journal of phytotherapy and phytopharmacology* vol. 51 (2018): 233-240. doi:10.1016/j.phymed.2018.10.014

[5] Glover, Louise E, and Sean P Colgan. "Hypoxia and metabolic factors that influence inflammatory bowel disease pathogenesis." *Gastroenterology* vol. 140,6 (2011): 1748-55. doi:10.1053/j.gastro.2011.01.056 https://www.ncbi.nlm.nih.gov/pmc/articles/PMC3093411/

[6] http://www.oxygenhealingtherapies.com/ozone_oxygen_therapies.html

[7] https://www.ozonetherapiesgroup.com/ozone-research/2019/10/19/oxidative-therapies-ozone-and-hydrogen-peroxide

[8] Maslennikov, O. V. et al. "Ozone Therapy in Practice", 2008 Russia https://www.absoluteozone.com/assets/ozone_therapy_in_practice.pdf

[9] https://www.austinozone.com/wp-content/uploads/GermanyGuidelines0309.pdf

[10] https://water-research.net/index.php/ozonation

EPILOGUE

Congratulations, my dear readers!

By now, you should have a better understanding of what it takes to stop IBD flare.

You are now clear about the root causes of IBD (Crohn's & colitis), and are now empowered with proven tools you need to heal your gut. This book is your trusted guide to wellness — if you made it this far, you already won half the battle. Now it's time for you to decide and act.

My promise to you: commit and complete this program and you will see results! You can truly heal. You are destined to enjoy a life of health, happiness, and freedom.

Your next step is to go to Chapter 7, and get started with preparing and organizing for the program. I recommend allocating enough free time (e.g., vacation time) for doing the program from beginning to end. At this stressful time in your life, if you want to get well fast, learn to put your health and your needs first.

I know if you follow this program diligently, you will be successful in FINALLY STOPPING YOUR IBD FLARES. Now, you have step-by-step instructions on how to do it properly and effectively!

My next book, Crohn's and Colitis Healing System™, describes in detail what should be done next to CREATE A SUPER HEALTHY GUT!

What you will learn in this new book

- How to identify hidden triggers that cause Crohn's & Colitis symptoms
- New, effective life-saving tips and modalities for ultimate CD & UC healing
- How to gain weight and remedy malnutrition by improving digestion and absorption
- Foods and common supplements you should avoid at all costs, and the reasons why
- A three-phase plan that helps you achieve the ultimate goal - long lasting remission

Remember, you are in control of your body and your destiny.

If this book has helped you stop your IBD flare and improved your quality of life, please let my team know at feedback@knowyourgut.com. We appreciate your feedback and gut healing testimonials.

You can, and you will, stop your flare. I believe in you! YOU must now believe in yourself!

Yours in health,
Galina Kotlyar, MS RD LDN
www.knowyourgut.com

Printed in the United States
by Baker & Taylor Publisher Services